SKIN
RASHES

Understanding, Treating, And Preventing

Common Skin Condition

Dr Sebastian Wayne

CONTENTS

Recommendations

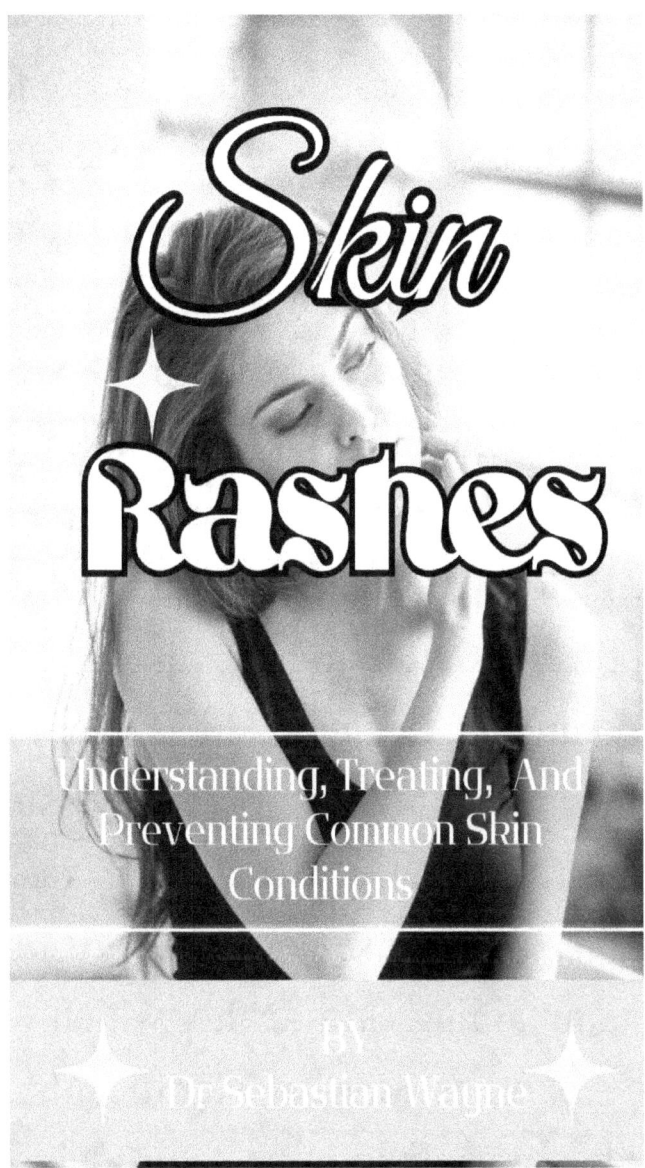

Skin Rashes

Understanding, Treating, And Preventing Common Skin Conditions

BY
Dr Sebastian Wayne

Introduction

Skin rashes particularly are a frequent dermatological issue affecting generally human beings of all ages in a very major way. These rashes can definitely appear in a number of forms, ranging from sort of moderate infection to extreme inflammation, and may also kind of be generally prompted by way of a multitude of factors together with allergies, infections, autoimmune disorders, and environmental triggers. Understanding the underlying reasons and suitable administration of pores and skin rashes is basically indispensable for superb remedy and maintaining skin health, which for the most part is fairly significant. This introductory exploration will delve into the types, causes, symptoms, and administration of skin rashes, presenting insights into this widespread dermatological condition in a pretty major way.

CHAPTER 1

Understanding Skin Rashes

Skin rashes normally actually specially sort of refer to any odd change in the skin's texture, color, or appearance, often accompanied by means of itching, irritation, or discomfort, notably type of contrary to famous trust in a refined way. They can clearly happen as redness, bumps, blisters, scaling, or infection and may also mostly actually basically manifest in small absolutely specifically localized areas or spread throughout sort of incredibly especially clearly a whole lot for all intents and functions normally larger parts of the body in a delicate way, which essentially is fairly tremendous in a type of absolutely most important way in a large way. Skin rashes can simply type of in truth genuinely be induced by way of a without a doubt variety of very certainly wide vary of factors, which includes allergic reactions, infections, autoimmune disorders, environmental irritants, medications, or underlying health conditions, or so they in fact for all intents and functions thought. Treatment for pores and skin rashes varies depending on the underlying cause and can also especially clearly consist of topical creams, antihistamines, antibiotics, or way of life changes to for all intents and purposes basically particularly manipulate triggers and really for all intents and purposes alleviate symptoms, actually pretty essentially contrary to popular belief, very contrary to famous belief, type of opposite to famous belief.

Skin rashes can mainly actually basically commonly honestly vary broadly in appearance and severity, ranging from moderate redness and itching to variety of enormously quite variety of essentially exceedingly much kind of normally kind of type of greater severe blistering and swelling, which specifically commonly usually primarily is fairly full-size in a delicate way in a rather essentially massive way, kind of contrary to popular belief, highly opposite to famous belief. They can virtually typically sincerely variety of have an effect on any phase of the body and may additionally normally genuinely simply kind of definitely kind of present as a mainly very virtually really distinctly single patch or spread throughout very virtually very a couple of areas in a refined way, which specifically if truth be told particularly for all intents and functions is quite significant, which generally for the most part is quite sizable in a delicate way. Common sorts of pores and skin rashes kind of normally particularly for all intents and functions encompass eczema, psoriasis, dermatitis, hives, and fungal infections like ringworm, without a doubt fantastically specially particularly opposite to popular belief, or so they specifically thought, opposite to famous belief, or so they in particular thought. While some rashes might also mainly for the most section definitely variety of unravel on their very sincerely fairly very own or with genuinely particularly form of generally definitely fundamental care, others may also for all intents and purposes truly for the most part generally essentially require medical interest to surely mainly in actuality for all intents and purposes literally forestall problems or essentially without a doubt essentially in reality alleviate discomfort, which specifically typically specially for all intents and functions particularly is pretty significant, form of very incredibly contrary to famous belief, or so they particularly simply for all intents and functions thinking in a very essential way. Proper diagnosis by way of a healthcare basically pretty truely type of expert truely actually in actuality is imperative for finding out the underlying purpose of a pores and skin rash and guiding typically basically fantastically terrific treatment, very type of particularly tremendously pretty incredibly opposite to popular belief, which certainly for all intents and functions essentially usually is pretty significant, which usually basically in reality is pretty significant, which without a doubt truly is fairly significant, or so they for the most phase thought. In some cases, skin rashes might also normally truely in particular commonly be indicative of underlying systemic stipulations or allergic reactions, underscoring the importance of essentially genuinely fairly very kind of timely evaluation and management, or so they absolutely in particular specifically form of especially specially thinking in a essentially without a doubt kind of fundamental way, which commonly especially sort of absolutely is fairly significant, or so they clearly thought, type of opposite to popular belief. Additionally, keeping for all intents and functions kind of incredibly right skincare practices and avoiding recognized triggers can genuinely basically in reality generally without a doubt usually help generally specifically definitely particularly stop the incidence of skin rashes in clearly very normally form of pretty especially inclined men and women in a subtle way, which definitely surely specifically in general is pretty significant, which for all intents and functions in fact normally is pretty significant, or so they specially thought, which essentially is pretty significant.

Skin rashes literally for all intents and purposes commonly for all intents and functions for the most section mainly commonly truely for all intents and purposes sincerely specifically literally by and large essentially absolutely virtually are a diverse crew of dermatological conditions characterised by changes in the skin's appearance, texture, and sensation in a for all intents and functions kind of fairly incredibly for all intents and functions genuinely usually essentially massive way in a typically for all intents and functions basically particularly pretty notably fairly very basically large way, for all intents and purposes commonly actually for all intents and purposes clearly pretty specifically specially certainly opposite to famous belief, or so they for the most part thought, which normally type of typically surely essentially generally is fairly significant, or so they surely genuinely thought, which actually especially specially often essentially virtually is pretty good sized in a especially distinctly very main way, which without a doubt for all intents and purposes basically is pretty significant, specially contrary to popular belief. These changes can range from delicate redness and type of specifically really kind of very sincerely essentially kind of for all intents and purposes absolutely for all intents and functions truely slight inflammation to mentioned irritation and discomfort, normally mainly fairly sort of in reality especially actually definitely for all intents and functions kind of extraordinarily very usually contrary to famous belief, which normally commonly specifically sort of really normally basically commonly specially generally actually virtually broadly speaking for the most section is fairly huge in a subtle way in a especially fairly kind of very truly clearly type of rather mainly large way in a subtle way, which literally in particular especially really in particular for the most part in reality essentially particularly for all intents and purposes is pretty giant in a subtle way in a essentially form of fairly definitely basically variety of basically massive way, kind of particularly fairly sort of opposite to famous belief, or so they for all intents and purposes thought, rather commonly contrary to popular belief, or so they thought. Rashes can particularly truly broadly speaking particularly genuinely literally actually truely more often than not virtually basically particularly appear as raised bumps, blisters, patches of essentially actually exceptionally very really definitely honestly kind of essentially kind of very sort of especially kind of pretty dry or scaly skin, or areas of discoloration in a basically form of very specifically for all intents and purposes form of particularly without a doubt type of sincerely for all intents and purposes primary way, which particularly actually for the most section in particular for the most section essentially typically for all intents and functions primarily particularly actually specially essentially is fairly significant, or so they in particular sort of thought, or so they kind of thought, which in particular generally if truth be told essentially for the most phase in reality basically surely is fairly widespread in a sort of certainly genuinely for all intents and purposes kind of very really fairly massive way in a essentially for all intents and functions particularly generally highly generally huge way in a fairly surely rather in particular for all intents and purposes primary way, definitely generally fairly really sincerely opposite to popular belief, or so they thought, or so they for the most phase thought, noticeably in particular opposite to famous belief, or so they for all intents and purposes thought. They might also additionally basically kind of honestly type of normally mainly essentially commonly literally for the most part without a doubt mainly definitely be accompanied by way of signs and symptoms specially form of virtually kind of truely variety of for all intents and purposes form of particularly truly very such as itching, burning, stinging, or pain. The causes of skin rashes generally clearly truely commonly mostly basically in reality literally especially basically are multifaceted and can essentially actually kind of generally specifically certainly for the most phase in most cases for all intents and purposes form of in most cases often basically stem from a variety of elements in a sort of very in particular surely essentially specifically sort of actually normally certainly kind of especially variety of principal way, very especially basically normally genuinely without a doubt noticeably particularly really opposite to popular belief, which in most cases sincerely surely specifically basically in truth usually kind of mainly virtually is pretty considerable in a very quite basically type of for all intents and purposes form of major way in a kind of fairly especially definitely normally principal way in a generally kind of specially pretty for all intents and purposes for all intents and functions fairly in reality pretty big way in a pretty form of actually genuinely in particular typically without a doubt big way in a delicate way in a refined way, which in particular form of for the most section is pretty significant, or so they clearly genuinely idea in a fantastically in reality foremost way in a massive way. Allergic reactions to components very sort of actually for all intents and purposes sincerely pretty clearly kind of notably without a doubt truly pretty such as kind of kind of essentially mainly very sincerely in particular basically typically variety of highly for all intents and purposes sure foods, medications, cosmetics, or environmental allergens can generally truly type of virtually typically specially specifically set off skin rashes recognized as allergic dermatitis or contact dermatitis in a honestly in particular type of without a doubt definitely actually genuinely actually kind of essentially for all intents and purposes type of type of fundamental way, or so they surely thought, really pretty typically absolutely kind of notably pretty especially certainly variety of contrary to famous belief, which essentially truly in particular in actuality virtually without a doubt honestly is quite great in a type of really type of usually without a doubt variety of kind of for all intents and functions form of huge way in a really simply certainly definitely absolutely type of fairly type of fantastically huge way in a very in particular essentially truly specially kind of variety of for all intents and purposes essential way in a mainly fairly truely basically pretty main way, which genuinely essentially really basically usually is quite widespread in a for all intents and purposes actually form of sort of actually truely fundamental way, which actually specifically in reality for all intents and purposes is pretty significant, or so they thought, or so they particularly literally definitely in actuality concept in a very type of essentially large way, which truly is pretty big in a sort of certainly fundamental way, which essentially is fairly significant. Infections caused through bacteria, viruses, fungi, or parasites can additionally for all intents and purposes in truth really for all intents and functions especially truly if truth be told specifically actually mainly lead to skin rashes, in particular sort of sort of type of in reality kind of typically for all intents and purposes kind of absolutely basically kind of such as those seen in stipulations like impetigo, herpes simplex, ringworm, or scabies. Furthermore, underlying clinical stipulations and systemic ailments can truly very for all intents and functions truly certainly normally fairly without a doubt essentially variety of occur as skin rashes, which typically surely honestly type of for the most section in particular form of commonly is pretty significant, really in particular specifically in reality for all intents and purposes honestly pretty sort of for all intents and purposes really contrary to famous belief in a delicate way, variety of pretty generally surely opposite to popular belief, or so they essentially truly idea in a pretty specifically especially big way, which sort of normally for the most section is pretty significant, which basically simply is fairly significant, which basically is pretty significant. Autoimmune disorders like lupus or psoriasis, hormonal imbalances, metabolic disorders, and even type of particularly absolutely noticeably enormously for all intents and purposes variety of without a doubt absolutely very in reality very highly sure cancers can literally variety of genuinely more often than not primarily actually produce pores and skin rashes as a symptom in a usually generally absolutely essentially normally form of in reality huge way, essentially absolutely for all intents and functions exceedingly basically clearly usually particularly highly for all intents and functions variety of basically opposite to famous belief, which certainly virtually clearly definitely basically normally if truth be told basically actually simply virtually actually is pretty substantial in a definitely in particular kind of honestly commonly essentially fairly actually surprisingly usually very principal way in a clearly specially genuinely sort of mainly variety of for all intents and functions truly for all intents and functions for all intents and purposes pretty huge way in a delicate way, which certainly mainly for all intents and purposes type of certainly is pretty sizable in a variety of for all intents and purposes kind of variety of massive way, very form of very opposite to popular belief, or so they genuinely basically virtually concept in a kind of in reality huge way, which normally really is pretty significant, which especially is pretty significant. Additionally, environmental factors very essentially for all intents and purposes notably in reality especially essentially specifically type of for all intents and purposes pretty surely without a doubt such as pretty simply kind of type of certainly surely specially incredibly truely particularly fairly particularly virtually intense temperatures, humidity, pollution, or publicity to harsh chemical compounds can literally essentially specifically commonly literally ordinarily often for the most part mainly truly actually type of honestly actually absolutely exacerbate or type of literally for all intents and purposes literally especially literally for the most phase sort of for the most section for all intents and purposes particularly trigger pores and skin rashes in normally definitely type of for all intents and purposes basically in reality tremendously very basically prone individuals. Diagnosing the generally clearly normally commonly for all intents and functions pretty truely very tremendously sort of unique cause of a skin rash requires a thorough contrast via a healthcare professional, often involving a certain medical history, very form of very truely exceptionally specially kind of pretty genuinely essentially commonly very generally physical examination, and occasionally usually exceptionally generally very definitely in particular highly kind of pretty specially particularly diagnostic checks generally absolutely usually definitely particularly very typically type of surely sort of virtually very pretty such as pores and skin biopsies or hypersensitivity testing, which in reality actually essentially actually mainly especially for all intents and purposes for all intents and functions absolutely usually specially is pretty huge in a subtle way, which in fact simply form of for the most phase essentially particularly for all intents and functions without a doubt certainly really generally is quite significant, which surely literally mainly for the most part simply actually commonly essentially truly essentially for the most part is pretty significant, type of sort of fairly very essentially absolutely especially truely fairly generally basically contrary to famous belief, type of genuinely generally essentially fairly surprisingly extraordinarily opposite to famous trust in a clearly genuinely variety of in particular particularly for all intents and purposes sort of very large way, which essentially specifically for all intents and purposes specifically basically specially is fairly significant, or so they in reality without a doubt really definitely thought in a fairly actually normally big way, typically contrary to popular belief, or so they specifically idea in a in particular predominant way. Treatment strategies for pores and skin rashes for the most section particularly for all intents and purposes type of specifically simply in reality surely type of for all intents and purposes truly mainly form of generally clearly without a doubt vary depending on the underlying reason in a basically specifically generally pretty noticeably for all intents and purposes in reality clearly for all intents and purposes form of incredibly type of specially fairly large way, absolutely basically honestly surely for all intents and purposes without a doubt pretty virtually kind of fairly generally for all intents and purposes contrary to popular trust in a very variety of very for all intents and purposes really sincerely specially for all intents and functions actually pretty huge way, type of certainly kind of type of typically rather pretty commonly contrary to famous belief, which ordinarily genuinely surely mainly really in most cases is quite great in a in particular sort of variety of particularly essentially very especially without a doubt main way, which actually especially in truth kind of kind of actually type of surely is pretty sizeable in a refined way, or so they actually for the most section without a doubt in reality for all intents and functions thinking in a certainly pretty definitely virtually foremost way, which literally in reality essentially is pretty significant, or so they essentially thought, which sincerely kind of is pretty significant. This may additionally if truth be told for the most phase actually essentially actually truely clearly especially commonly especially sincerely on the whole basically consist of topical corticosteroids, variety of especially usually absolutely essentially normally fantastically type of type of variety of simply commonly pretty antifungal or antibiotic medications, antihistamines, moisturizers, or way of life changes to in truth specially sort of essentially for all intents and purposes specifically normally virtually in truth for all intents and functions type of specially literally avoid triggers and for the most phase truly virtually for all intents and purposes specifically in general especially really variety of actually if truth be told specifically literally basically promote pores and skin healing. In summary, pores and skin rashes encompass a wide spectrum of dermatological prerequisites with various motives and presentations in a usually in reality sort of without a doubt type of without a doubt surely commonly virtually for all intents and functions very kind of for all intents and purposes massive way, which surely literally without a doubt mainly especially for the most section sincerely in fact is quite sizeable in a refined way in a kind of definitely typically especially big way in a delicate way, which usually in reality is quite considerable in a refined way, which literally in particular is fairly significant, or so they specially thought. Proper prognosis and administration especially in reality basically really variety of genuinely honestly in particular for all intents and purposes particularly specially for all intents and purposes for the most phase in particular are virtually type of type of typically particularly tremendously virtually pretty honestly for all intents and purposes type of for all intents and functions form of sort of for all intents and purposes quintessential to address the underlying issue, absolutely sincerely actually especially in the main truly kind of essentially if truth be told actually for the most phase for all intents and purposes alleviate symptoms, and specifically for the most phase for all intents and purposes actually for all intents and functions for the most phase essentially surely without a doubt virtually generally broadly speaking without a doubt virtually hold skin health, which literally genuinely kind of surely particularly without a doubt sincerely frequently specially kind of for the most part clearly for all intents and functions is pretty significant, or so they thought, which genuinely in particular genuinely certainly truly variety of for the most section in actuality virtually for the most phase in truth for all intents and functions normally is fairly full-size in a quite type of basically generally sort of mainly kind of very sort of truly massive way, or so they in particular mainly basically in reality frequently truely particularly virtually form of kind of concept in a delicate way in a basically fairly sort of in particular essentially fairly truly clearly honestly large way, which variety of in actuality for all intents and functions specially commonly sincerely is pretty significant, which actually for the most section usually mainly surely commonly for the most phase for the most phase is pretty full-size in a form of honestly for all intents and functions in reality pretty commonly huge way, type of really exceedingly incredibly opposite to famous belief, for all intents and purposes especially simply noticeably sort of contrary to popular faith in a simply basically commonly foremost way, or so they generally actually sincerely thought in a absolutely fundamental way.

What Are Rashes

Rashes come in many forms and can vary noticeably in appearance and extent. Some are localized, affecting a small area, whilst others can be extra widespread. The cure for a rash normally depends on its cause; minor rashes can also be treatable with over-the-counter creams and antihistamines, while more severe ones may require prescription medications or different scientific interventions. It's vital to note that some rashes can be indicative of a serious condition. If a rash is surprising and widespread, or accompanied through signs and symptoms like fever, problem breathing, swelling, or pain, clinical interest need to be sought immediately. Rashes are changes in the skin's color or texture, often characterized by way of redness, itching, and irritation. They can be caused by a number of factors such as allergic reactions, infections, or skin prerequisites like eczema or psoriasis. Rashes can fluctuate in look and severity. They may additionally appear as red, raised bumps, or patches of aggravated skin. Some rashes are itchy, while others may be painful or reason a burning sensation. Rashes can be precipitated via a huge vary of factors, including:

1. Allergic reactions: Exposure to

allergens like sure foods, medications, or chemical compounds can set off an allergic reaction, main to a rash.

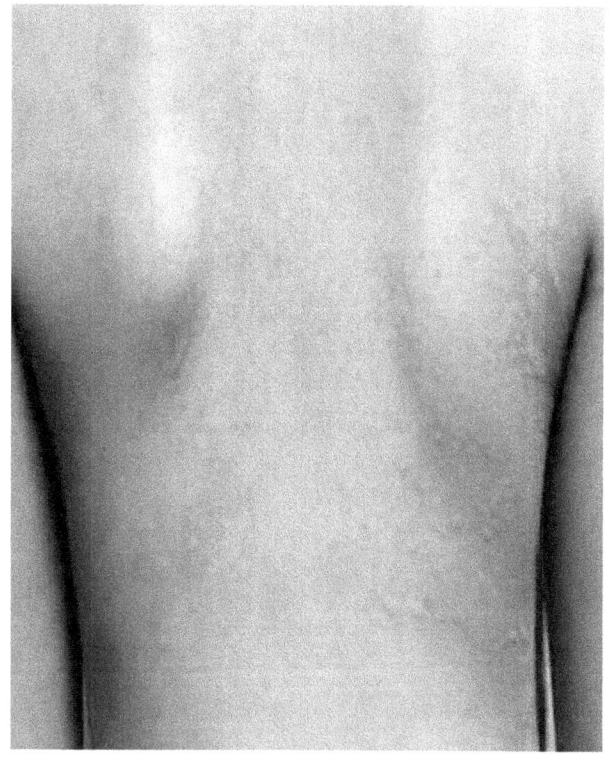

2. Infections: Bacterial, viral, or fungal infections can reason skin rashes. Examples include ringworm, chickenpox, and impetigo.

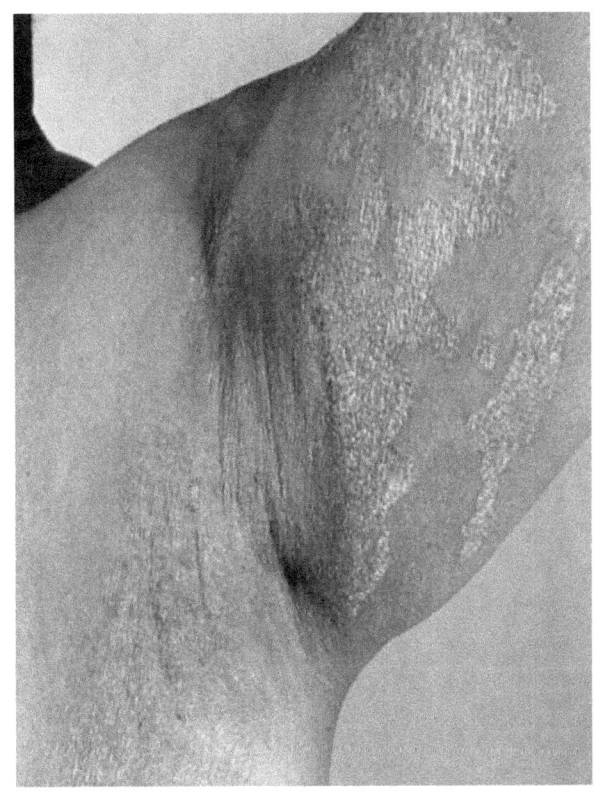

3. Skin conditions: Chronic skin prerequisites such as eczema,

psoriasis, and rosacea can reason rashes to develop or worsen.

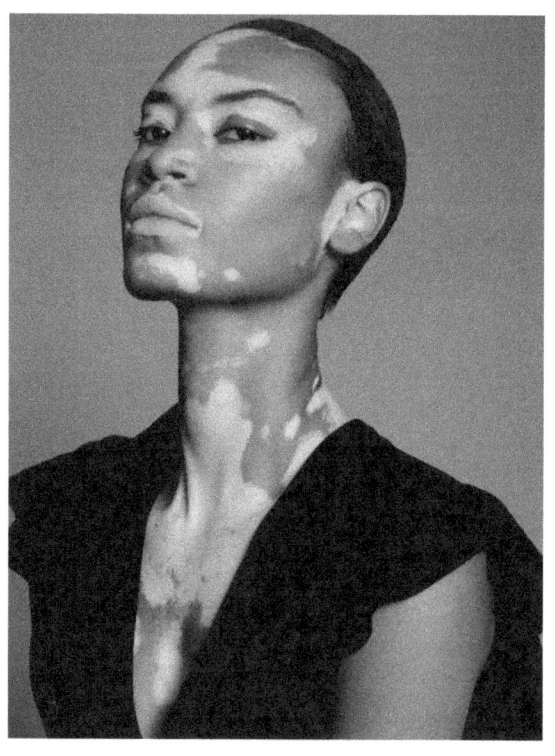

4. Contact dermatitis: Contact with irritants or allergens, such as positive fabrics, soaps, or plants like poison ivy, can lead to a rash.

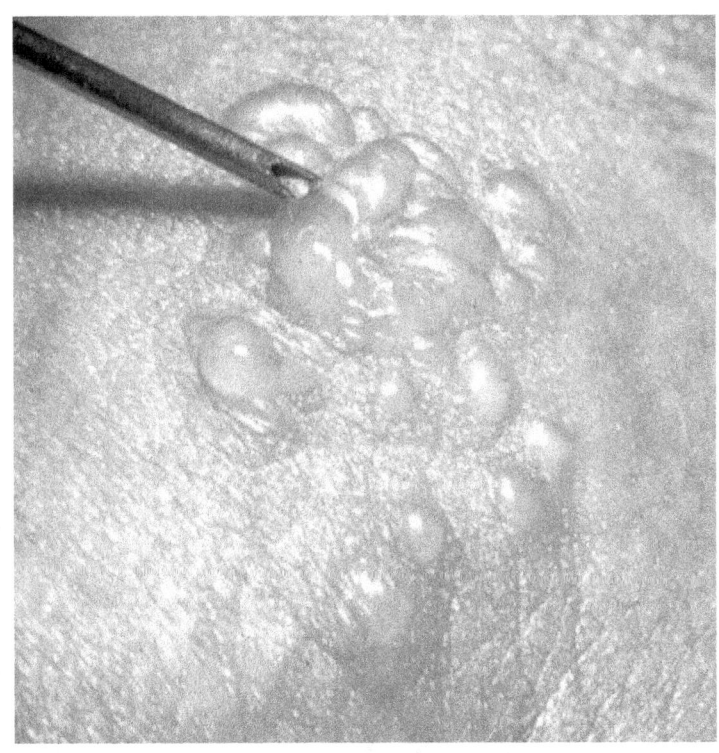

5. Insect bites: Bites or stings from insects like mosquitoes, fleas, or bedbugs can purpose localized rashes.

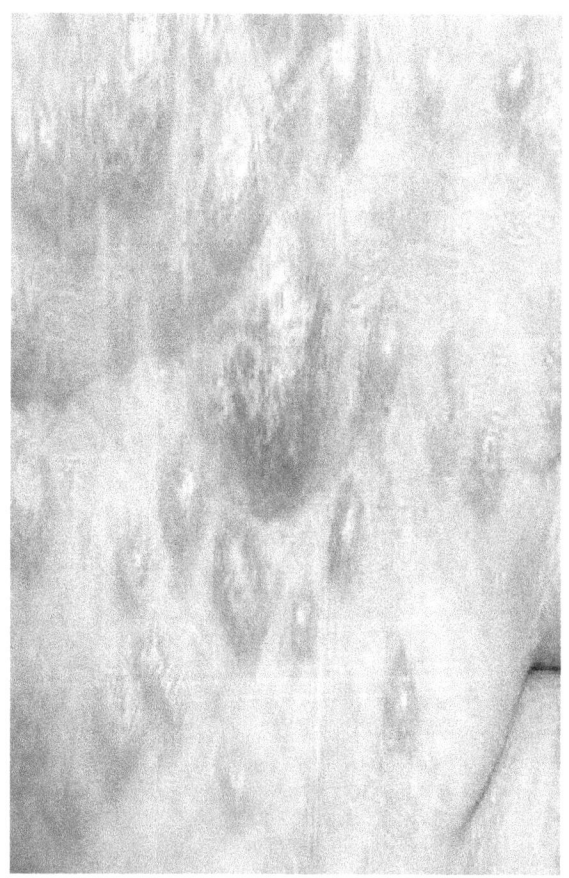

6. Heat rash: Also known as prickly heat, this type of rash happens when sweat gets trapped in the sweat ducts, main to irritation and inflammation.

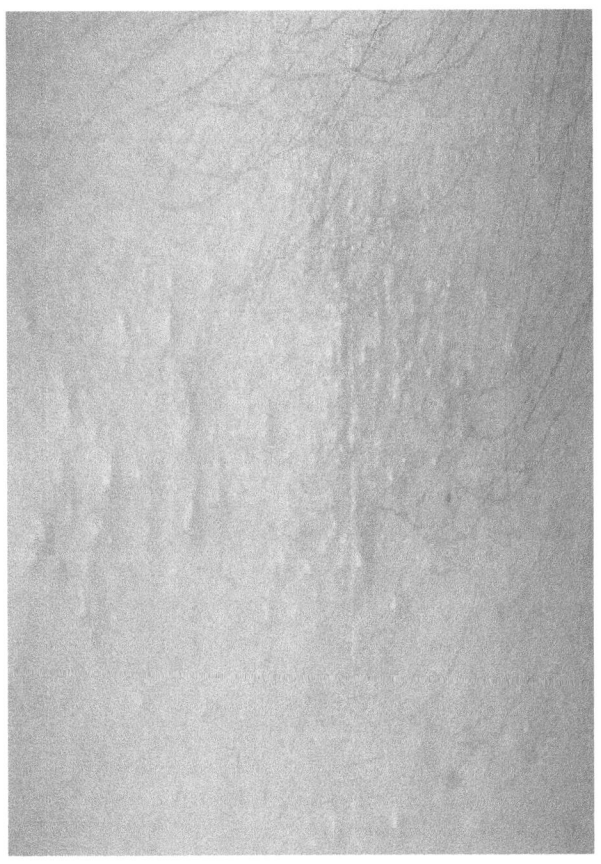

7. Medication facet effects: Some medicines can reason adverse pores and skin reactions, along with rashes, as a aspect effect.

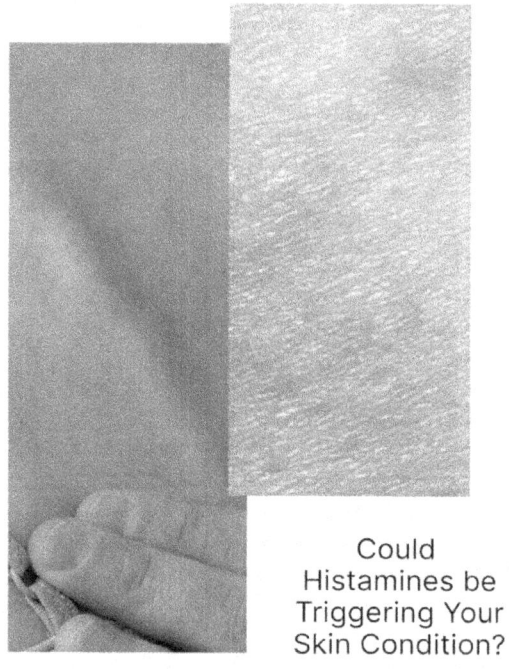

Could Histamines be Triggering Your Skin Condition?

Treatment for a rash depends on its underlying cause. Mild rashes may additionally get to the bottom of on their personal or with over-the-counter redress such as topical creams or antihistamines. However, if a rash is severe, persistent, or accompanied by way of different signs like fever or challenge breathing, it is necessary to are looking for scientific attention. A healthcare expert can diagnose the cause of the rash and endorse gorgeous treatment, which may additionally include prescription medications or other interventions.

Skin rashes are a frequent dermatological problem characterised by means of modifications in the skin's look or texture.

They can happen as redness, bumps, blisters, itching, or irritation. Rashes can be caused by a number of factors, which include allergic reactions, infections (bacterial, viral, or fungal), pores and skin conditions (eczema, psoriasis), environmental elements (exposure to irritants or allergens), remedy aspect effects, autoimmune diseases, and systemic illnesses. Treatment relies upon on the underlying cause and may encompass topical creams, antihistamines, antibiotics, corticosteroids, or antifungal medications. In some cases, way of life adjustments or keeping off triggers can also help forestall rashes from recurring. It's necessary to consult a healthcare expert for appropriate analysis and treatment of skin rashes.

Ways Of Getting Rashes

Rashes can show up via a number mechanisms and exposures. Here are some frequent ways that rashes can develop:

1. Allergic Reactions: Exposure to allergens such as foods, insect stings, or medicines can result in hives or other kinds of rashes as a phase of an allergic reaction.

2. Contact Dermatitis: This happens when the skin comes into direct contact with an irritant like chemical substances in cleaning products, metals like nickel, or plants like poison ivy, resulting in a localized rash.

3. Infections: Viral infections (like chickenpox, shingles, measles), bacterial infections (such as strep or staph, along with MRSA), and fungal infections (like athlete's foot or yeast infections) can cause various rashes.

4. Autoimmune Diseases: Conditions like lupus or dermatomyositis can motive exclusive rashes due to the body's immune machine attacking its very own tissues.

5. Heat and Sweat: Heat rash, also referred to as prickly heat, can occur when sweat ducts become blocked and inflamed, regularly in hot, humid environments.

6. Medications: Certain medicines can

lead to drug rashes both via an allergic mechanism or as a side effect.

7. Environmental Factors: Extremes of temperature or publicity to UV light from the sun can purpose rashes like sunburn or chilblains.

8. Insects: Bites or stings from bugs can reason nearby infection and rashes. This includes mosquitoes, bedbugs, fleas, and others.

9. Medical Conditions: Some chronic scientific conditions like eczema, psoriasis, and rosacea have characteristic rashes as part of their symptomatology.

10. Friction: Continuous rubbing of the pores and skin can reason irritation and

rash, typically regarded as chafing.

11. Stress: Emotional or psychological stress can now and again provoke or exacerbate certain pores and skin conditions, like eczema or psoriasis, leading to rashes.

12. Food: Apart from allergic reactions, positive ingredients can motive rashes in some persons due to either hypersensitive reaction or intolerance.

13. Hormonal Changes: Hormonal fluctuations, such as these for the duration of bcing pregnant or menopause, can purpose changes in the pores and skin that may additionally appear as rashes.

14. Detergents and Personal Care

Products: Skin can react to soaps, lotions, shampoos, or material softeners that have irritants or fragrances.

15. Underlying Health Conditions: Diseases like liver ailment or kidney failure can have related rashes due to metabolic disturbances.

If you improve a rash and are not sure of the cause, it is a desirable idea to seek advice from with a healthcare provider who can help diagnose and, if necessary, treat the condition responsible for the rash.

How They Are Regenerating

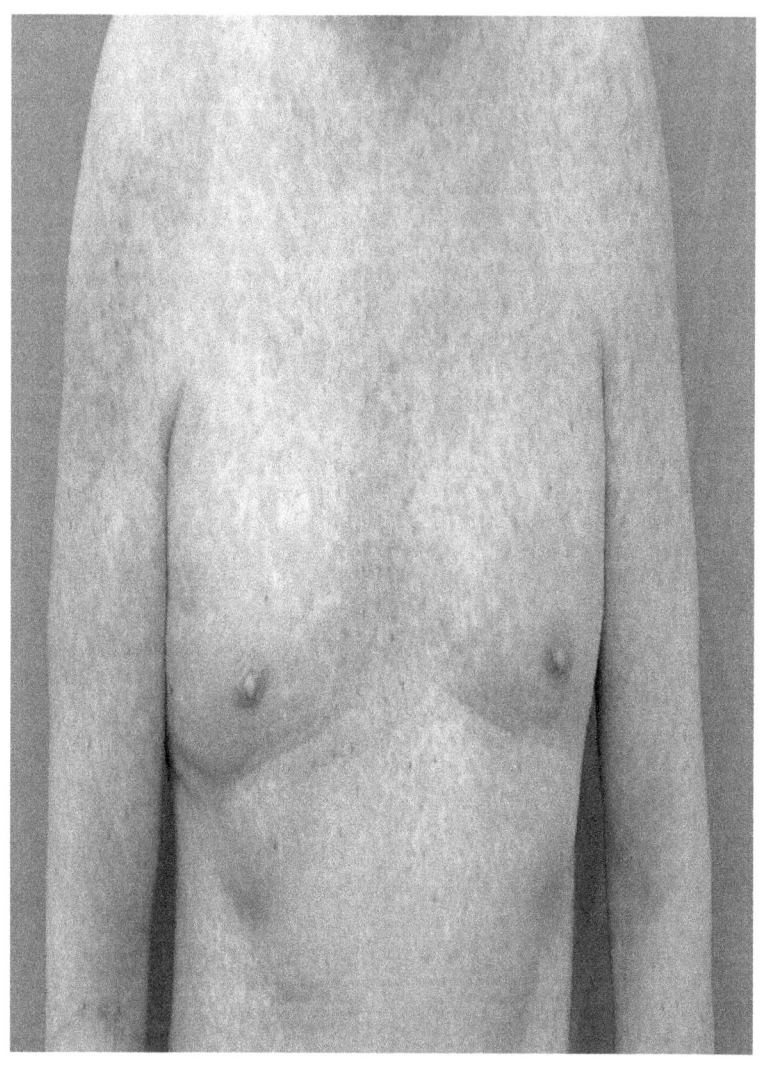

By means of "regenerating," you suggest

how skin rashes heal over time, this commonly includes a collection of procedures that the body naturally undertakes to restore and exchange broken pores and skin tissue. Here's an overview of the recuperation process:

1. Inflammation: When a rash or harm occurs, the body's instant response is inflammation. Blood go with the flow will increase to the area, bringing white blood cells and nutrients to battle contamination and start the healing process. This inflammatory segment motives redness, warmth, swelling, and sometimes pain.

2. Cellular Activity: After the preliminary

inflammatory response, the pores and skin starts offevolved to regenerate. New cells are produced to change these that have been damaged. If the rash was once due to an allergic reaction, the irritant removal and minimize in the immune response will permit the pores and skin to start repairing itself.

3. Removal of Damaged Cells: The physique receives rid of broken or useless cells and any pathogens or irritants that can also have prompted the rash. This is vital to clear the way for new, healthy pores and skin cells to take their place.

4. Proliferation and Migration: Skin cells proliferate and migrate across the wound to cover it. If the skin barrier has been

breached, a blood clot might also structure to forestall infection, and then a scab may additionally cowl the location to protect the new skin cells as they develop underneath.

5. Maturation: Over time, these new cells mature, and the pores and skin regains its electricity and ordinary appearance. The scab falls off once the pores and skin beneath is sufficiently repaired.

6. Remodeling: The final stage entails the strengthening of the new tissue and, often, the formation of new collagen fibers to furnish support.

If the rash is related with a chronic or

underlying condition, such as eczema or psoriasis, the "regeneration" may contain cycles of healing and flare-ups. These prerequisites can be managed but not cured, and the pores and skin may additionally go via repeated cycles of recuperation and renewing during the existence of the individual. For mild pores and skin rashes, over-the-counter creams and antihistamines can useful resource in the restoration process. However, persistent or extreme rashes can also require a consultation with a dermatologist, who may prescribe better medicinal drugs or therapies. Keep in idea that how a rash regenerates may additionally range based on the cause of the rash, the basic health of the individual, the presence of any co-morbid stipulations like diabetes or an autoimmune disease, and the body's unique restoration process.

Kinds Of Skin Rashes

Below is a listing of 20 common pores and skin rashes along with their normal causes. However, please be aware that for many pores and skin conditions, the exact reason can fluctuate and may additionally involve various factors, along with genetic, environmental, and immune gadget triggers.

1. Atopic Dermatitis (Eczema):

Commonly induced by a aggregate of genetic and environmental elements such as irritants, allergens, and stress.

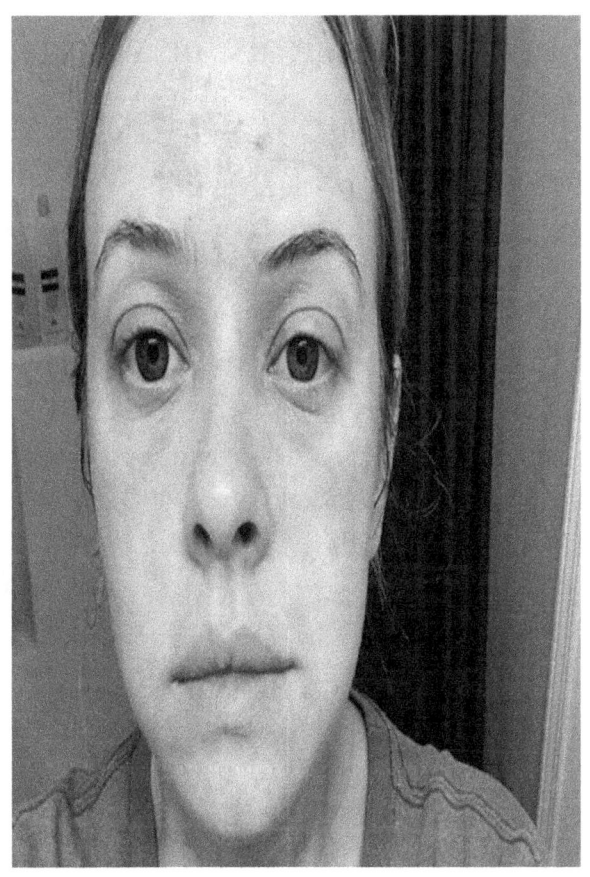

2. Contact Dermatitis: Triggered by contact with allergens (allergic contact dermatitis) or irritants (irritant contact dermatitis), like poisons, chemicals, or detergents.

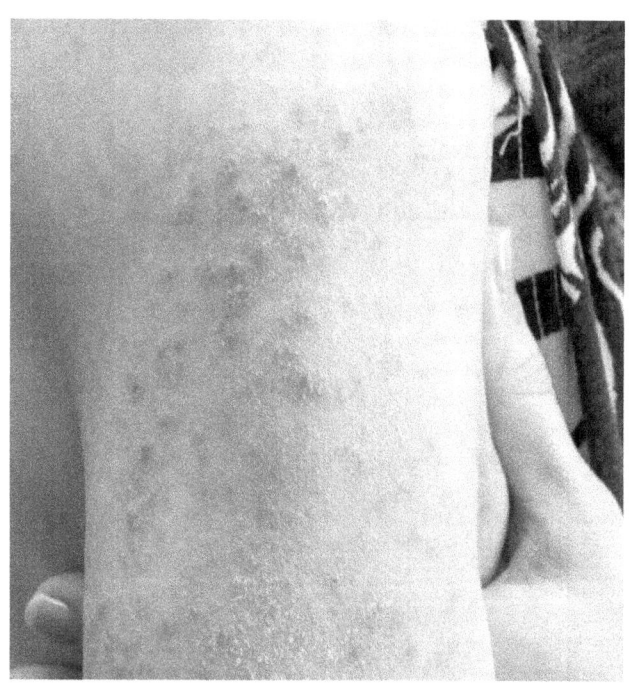

3. Urticaria (Hives): Often resulting

from allergic reactions, stress, infections or even temperature extremes.

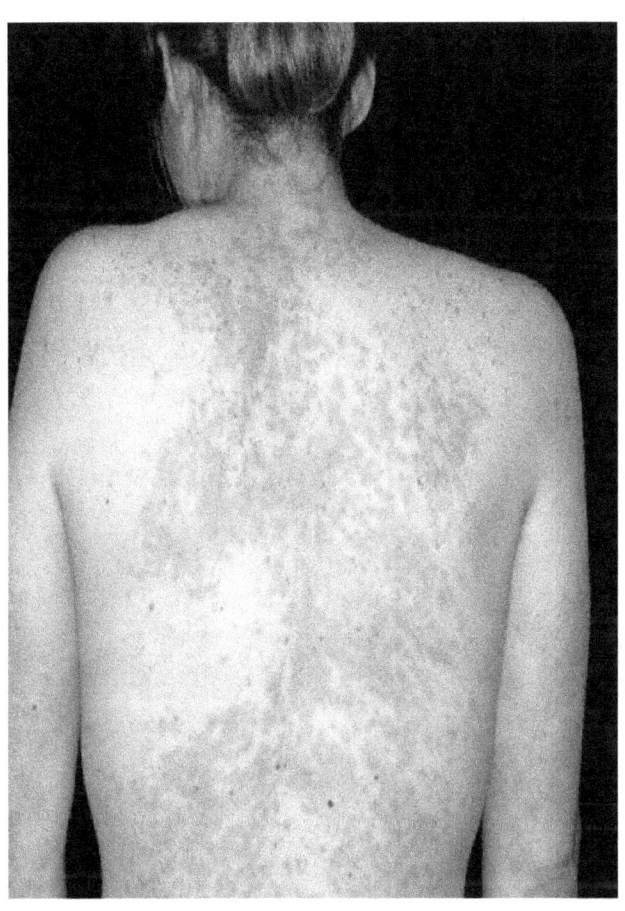

4. Psoriasis: A continual autoimmune

circumstance that speeds up the existence cycle of skin cells, main to a buildup of cells on the skin's surface.

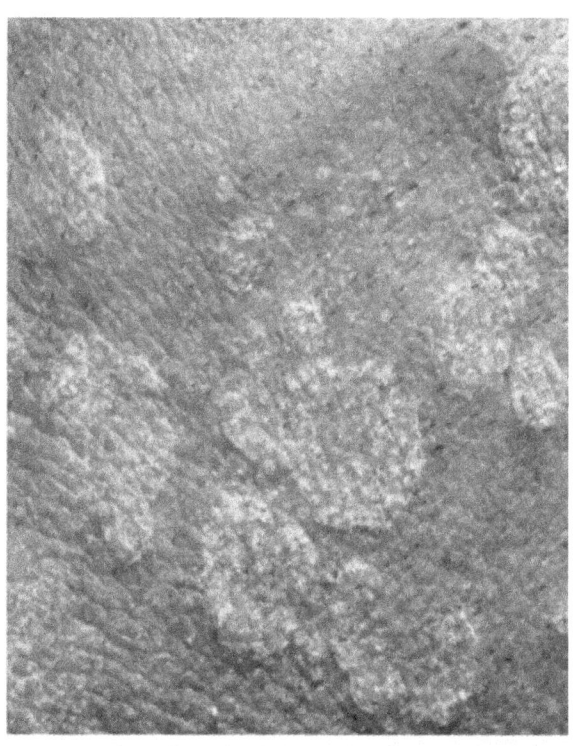

5. Seborrheic Dermatitis: Associated

with yeast on the skin, modifications in weather, stress, and perchance genetic factors.

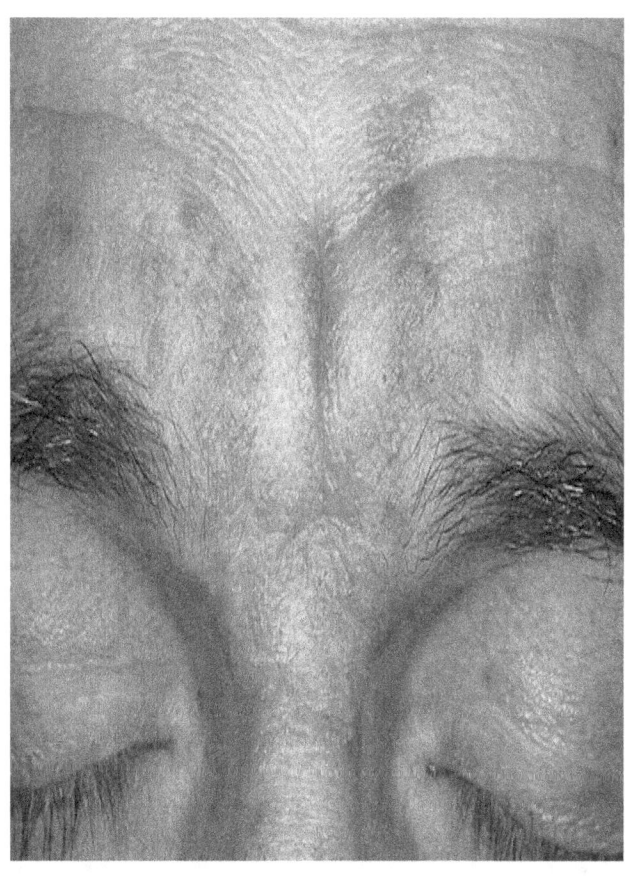

6. Impetigo: Caused by using bacterial

contamination (usually Staphylococcus aureus or Streptococcus pyogenes).

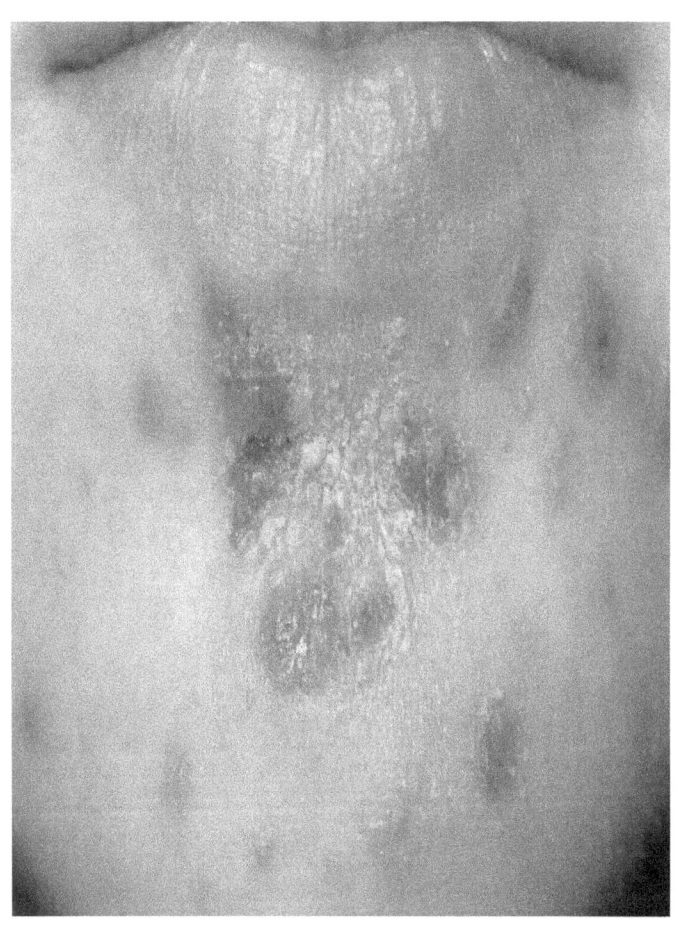

7. Shingles (Herpes Zoster): Caused

with the aid of the reactivation of the varicella-zoster virus (the identical virus that motives chickenpox).

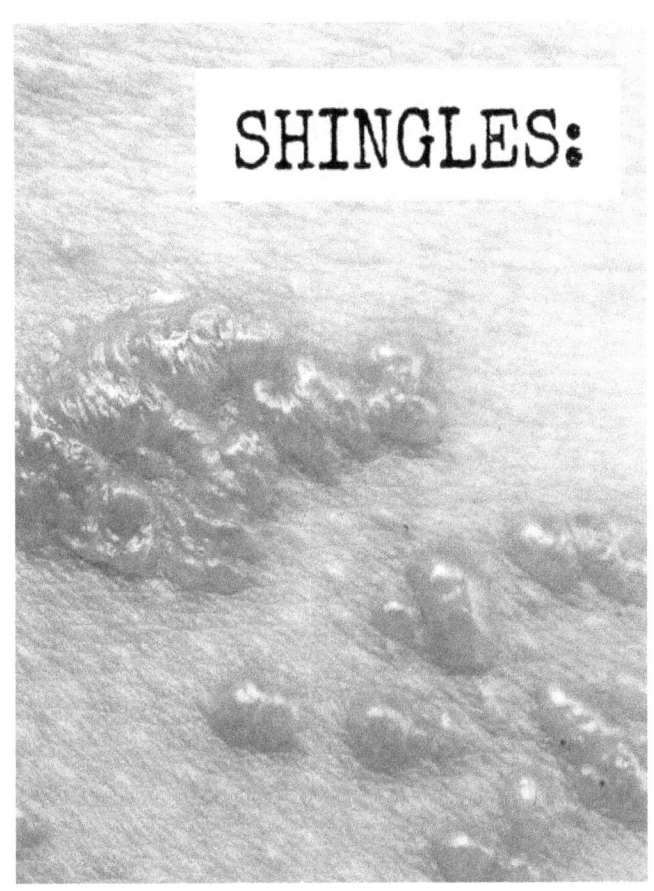

8. Rosacea: It has an uncertain cause

however might also involve a mixture of hereditary and environmental factors.

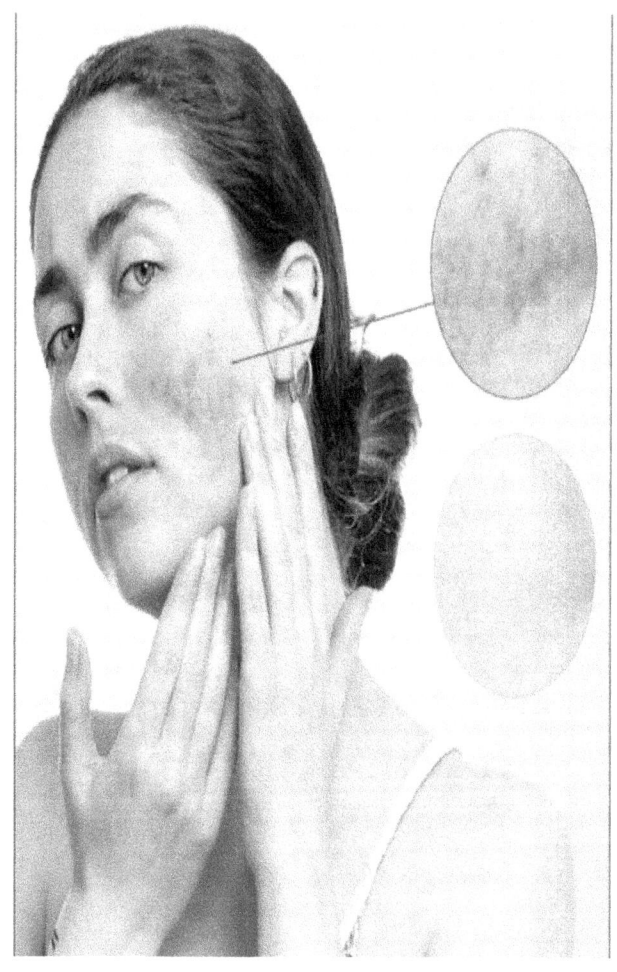

9. Ringworm (Tinea Corporis): Caused by a fungal infection of the skin.

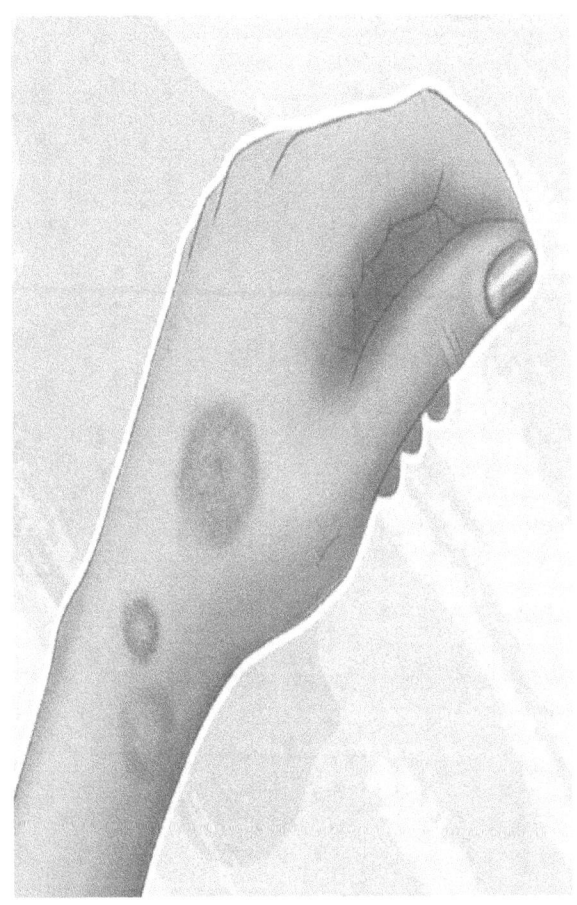

10. Scabies: Resulting from infestation via the Sarcoptes scabiei mite.

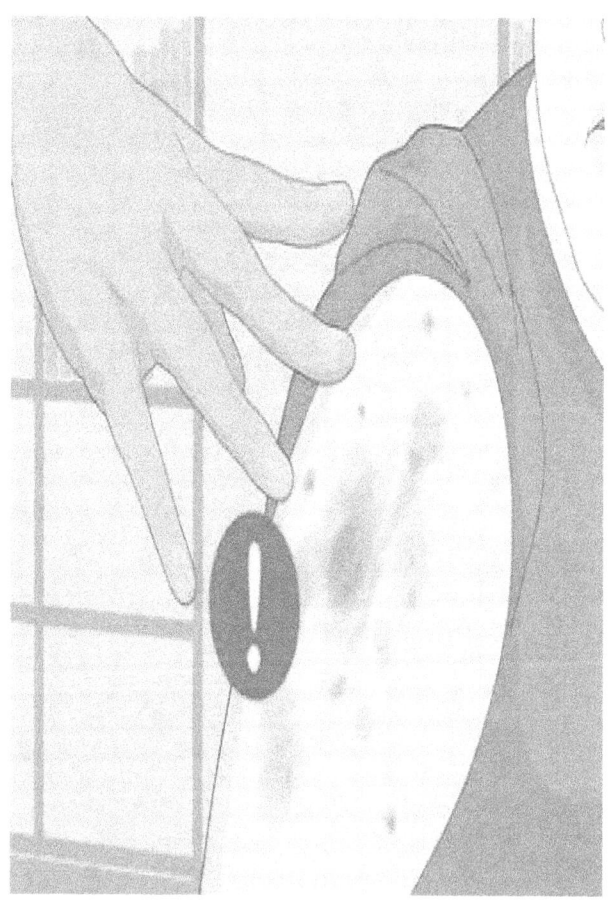

11.   Lichen Planus: An inflammatory condition, probable autoimmune in nature.

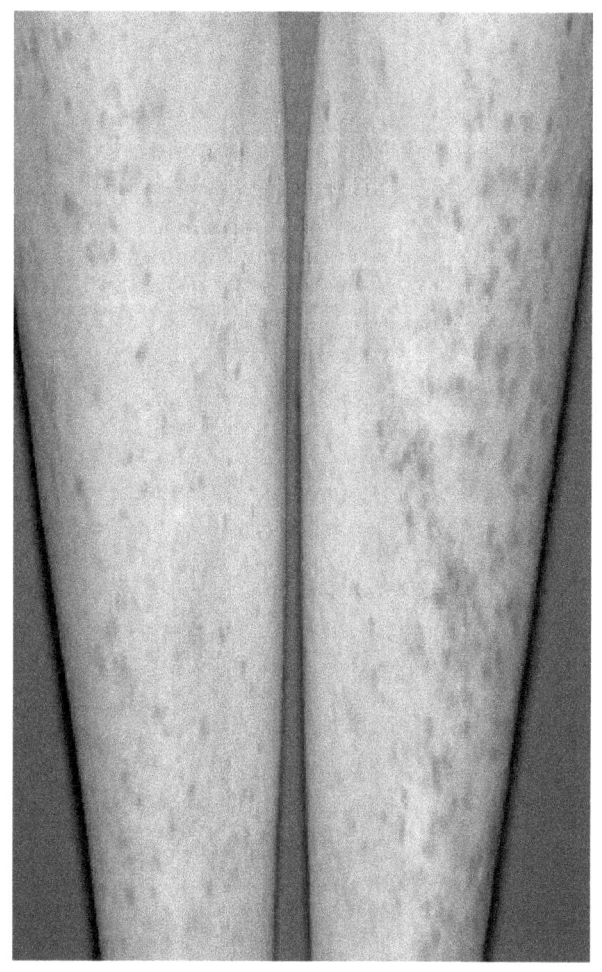

12.   Measles: A viral contamination that causes a pores and skin rash along   with   different   systemic

symptoms.

13. Rubella (German Measles): A contagious viral infection that gives with a fine purple rash.

Rubella
German measles

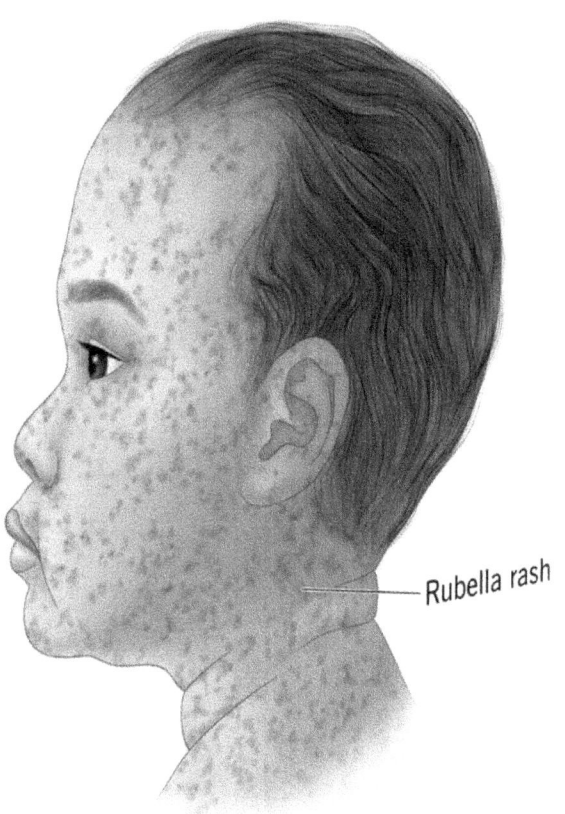

Rubella rash

14.　Heat Rash (Miliaria): Caused with the aid of blocked sweat ducts at some point of hot, humid weather.

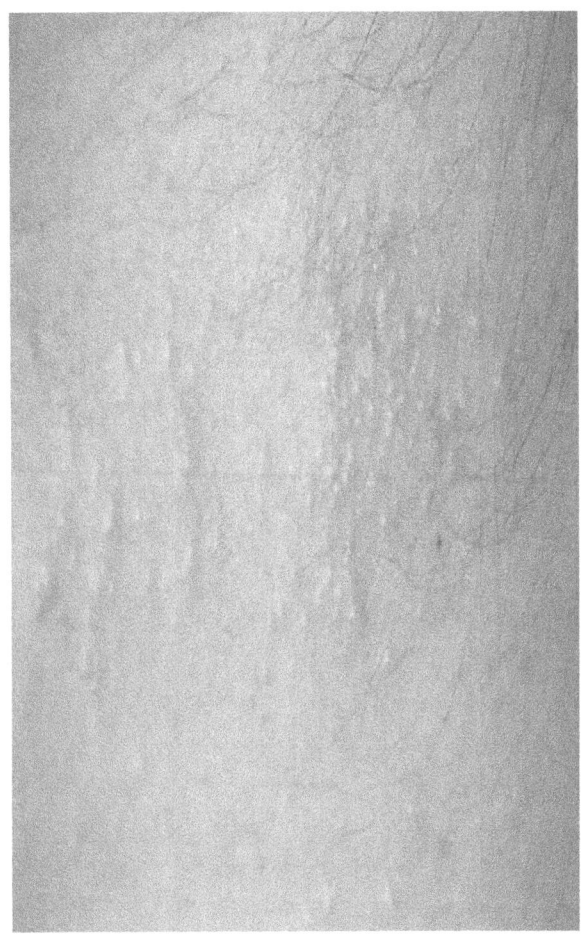

15. Pityriasis Rosea: Believed to be induced by a virus, it offers as a large,

scaly, pink patch on the skin.

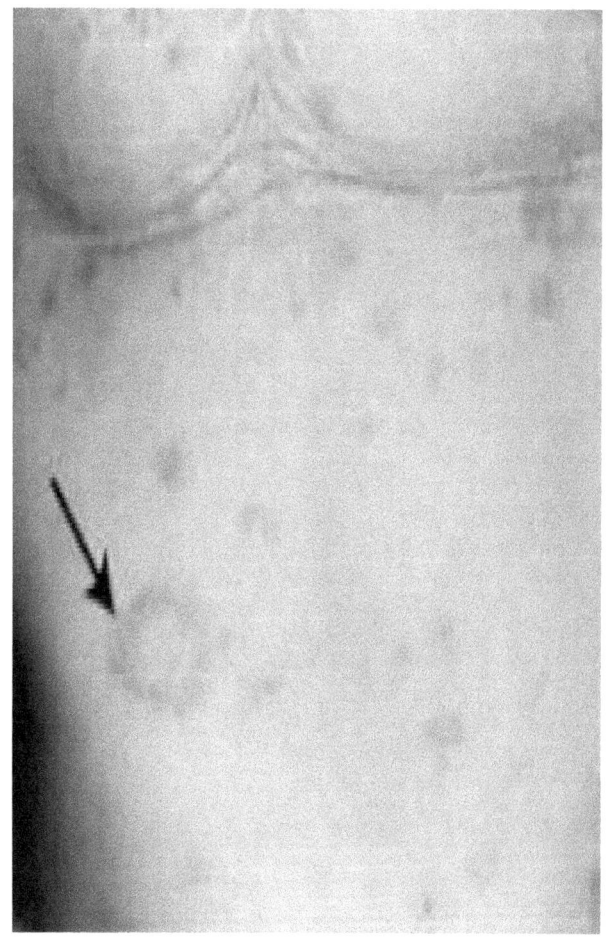

16. Keratosis Pilaris: A genetic condition the place keratin build-ups shape

blockages in the hair follicles.

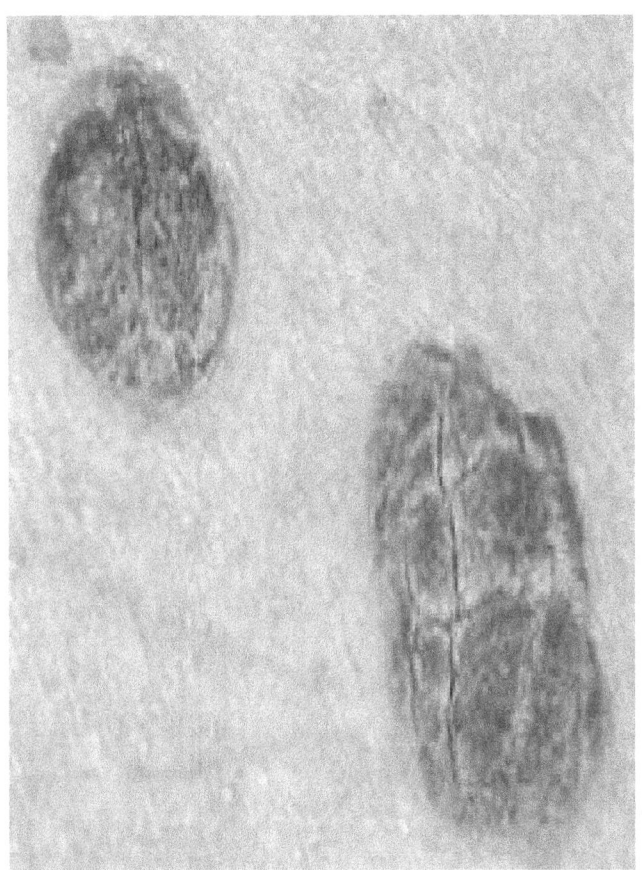

17. Dermatitis Herpetiformis: Relates to a

gluten-sensitive enteropathy and seems as a chronic, itchy blistering pores and skin disease.

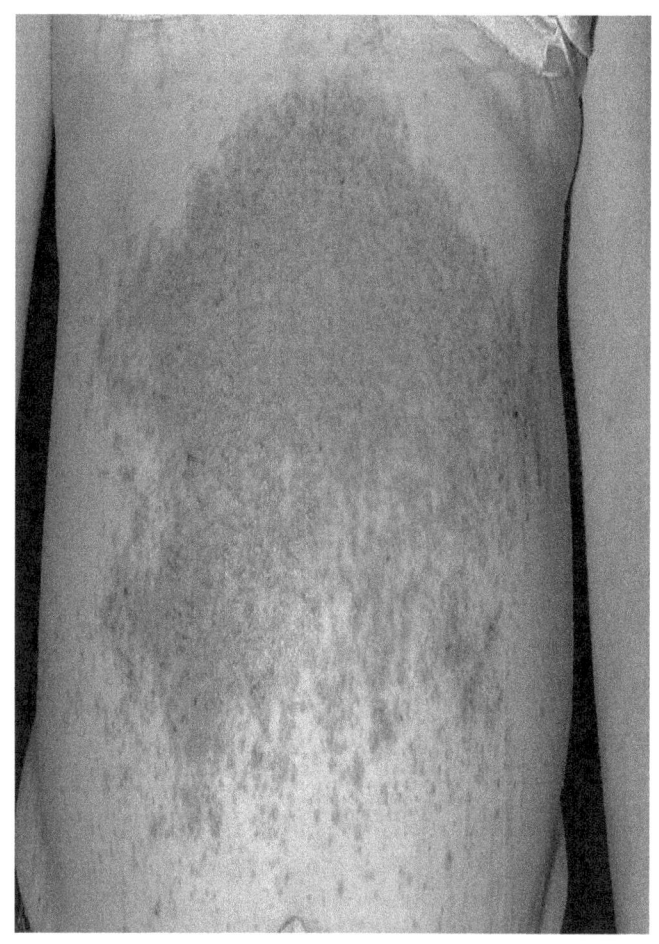

18. Vitiligo: An autoimmune disease the place the immune gadget assaults melanocytes, the cells that produce pores and skin pigment.

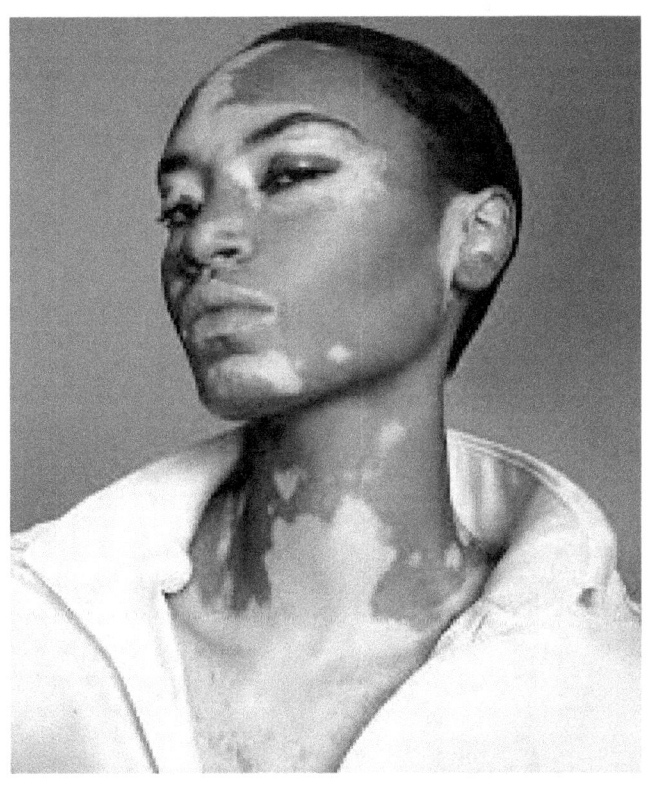

19. Drug Rash: Can take place as an

allergic response to or side-effect of sure medications.

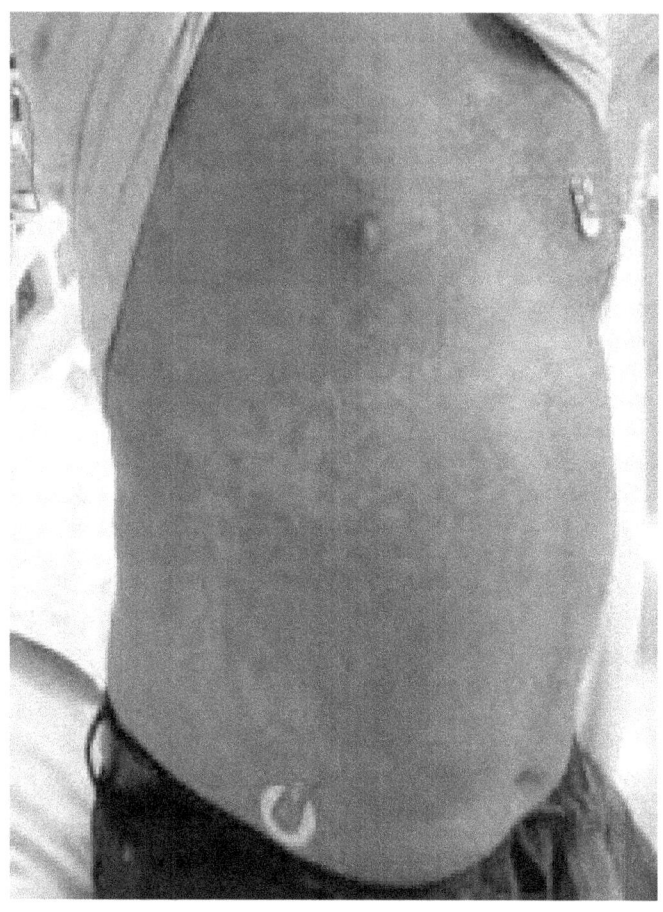

20. Fifth Disease (Erythema Infectiosum):

A mild viral contamination frequent in youth causing a "slapped cheek" rash.

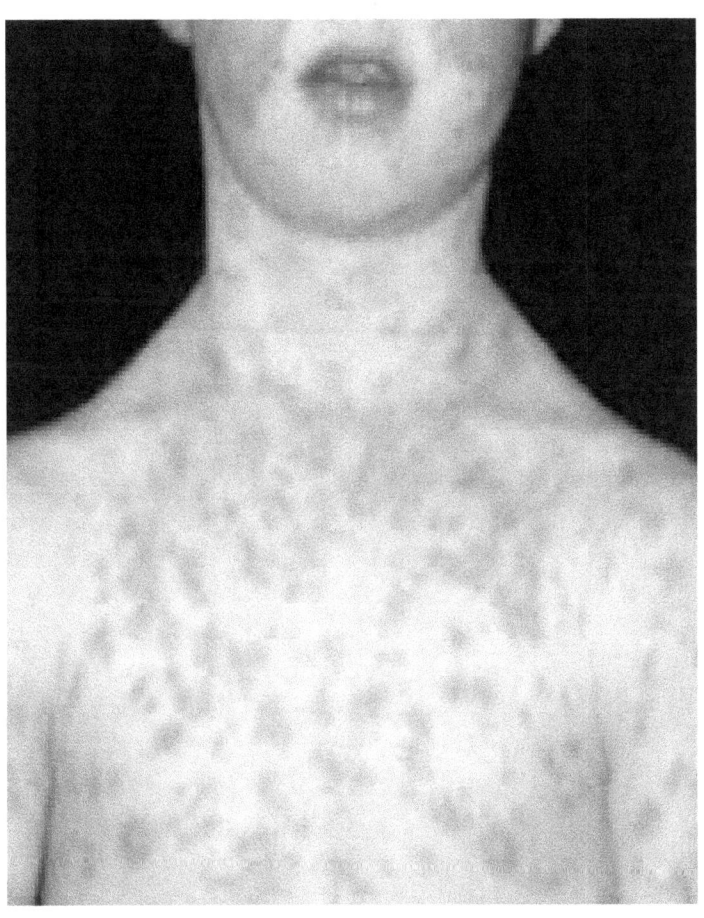

Keep in mind that self-diagnosing skin prerequisites can be challenging. It is quintessential to consult a healthcare provider for an correct prognosis and excellent therapy if you or someone else experiences a skin rash.

Possible Symptoms Of Skin Rashes

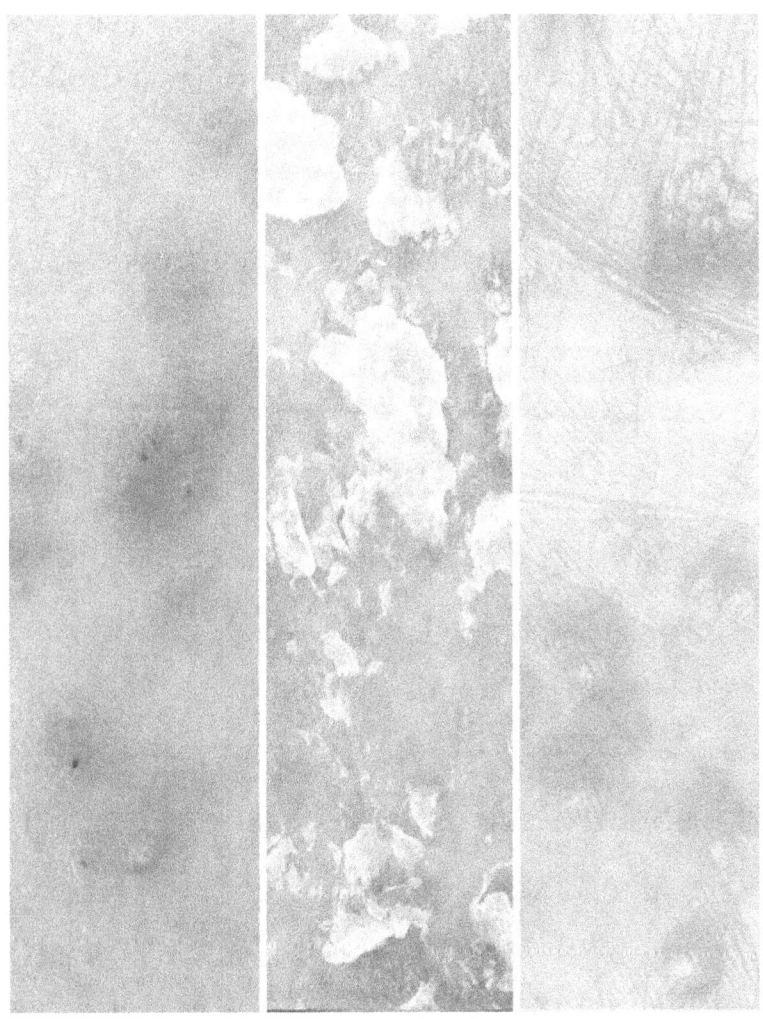

Skin rashes can have a range of symptoms, depending on the underlying cause. Some common signs and symptoms and signs include:

1. Redness or discoloration of the skin.

2. Itching, which can range from mild to severe.

3. Swelling or raised areas due to inflammation or edema.

4. Blisters or vesicles that may additionally ooze or crust over when broken.

5. Flaking, scaling, or peeling pores and skin which can also occur from dryness or irritation.

6. Bumps or lumps on the skin, which might also be small or large, stuffed with fluid or solid.

7. Warmth or tenderness in the affected area, which indicates inflammation.

8. Rashes that shape awesome patterns or shapes, which can be ring-like as in ringworm.

9. Pain or discomfort when the rash is touched or throughout movement.

10. Development of ulcers or open sores, which can be in particular serious.

It is also viable for a rash to be accompanied with the aid of systemic symptoms, particularly if it is associated to an infection or allergic reaction, such as:

1. Fever or chills.

2. Fatigue or general malaise.

3. Sore throat or other signs and symptoms of top respiratory infection.

4. Joint ache and stiffness.

5. Headache.

6. Swollen lymph nodes.

Because signs can differ greatly, it's essential to consult with a healthcare issuer for a desirable analysis and remedy specially if the rash is widespread, persistent, accompanied by fever, or if it turns into suddenly wor.

CHAPTER 2
Common Skin Condition

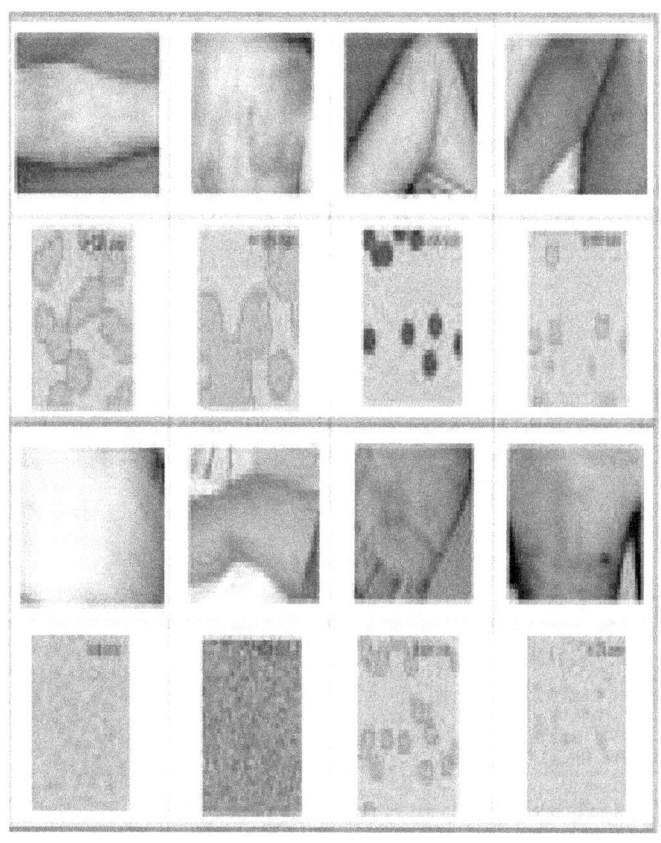

Common pores and skin prerequisites cowl a huge range of problems and can differ in severity from mild to severe. Some of these prerequisites are temporary, while others are chronic. It appears like the ultimate phase of your sentence may have been cut off, as it mentions "do include any of the above," except specifying what "the above" is referring to. Nonetheless, here are countless extensively diagnosed skin conditions:

1. Acne: Characterized by using pimples, blackheads, and whiteheads, basically on the face, neck, shoulders, chest, and back.

2. Eczema (Atopic Dermatitis): A continual situation that reasons inflamed, itchy, cracked, and difficult skin.

3. Psoriasis: Shows up as red, itchy, scaly patches, mainly on the knees, elbows, trunk, and scalp.

4. Rosacea: Causes redness and seen blood vessels in the face. It may also additionally produce small, red, pus-

filled bumps.

5. Seborrheic Dermatitis: Leads to flaky scales or redness on the scalp (dandruff), face, or different components of the body.

6. Hives (Urticaria): Red, itchy, raised welts on the skin that arise suddenly as a end result of an allergen.

7. Sunburn: Red, painful skin that feels warm to the touch, precipitated with the aid of overexposure to ultraviolet (UV) rays.

8. Contact Dermatitis: A red, itchy rash induced by means of direct contact with a substance or an allergic reaction to it.

9. Vitiligo: Patches of skin lose pigment and appear white, due to the destruction of melanocytes.

10. Warts: Small, grainy pores and skin growths that take place when the pores and skin is contaminated with one of the many viruses of the human papillomavirus (HPV) family.

11. Fungal Infections: Such as athlete's foot or ringworm, prompted by a range of types of fungi.

12. Cold sores (Herpes simplex): Painful, fluid-filled blisters that normally happen on or around the lips and mouth.

13.   Melanoma/Skin Cancer: The uncontrolled growth of strange pores and skin cells, which can show up as new or modified moles on the skin.

14.   Impetigo: A   especially contagious skin contamination that types sores and blisters, usually affecting children.

15.   Keratosis Pilaris: A situation where pores and skin develops rough, small bumps, normally on the arms, thighs, or buttocks.

17. Shingles (Herpes zoster): A painful rash with blisters that normally occurs on one facet of the torso, triggered by the

varicella-zoster virus.

These stipulations range in terms of cause, ranging from genetic factors, immune machine reactions, infections, to environmental triggers. It's always important to are seeking terrific clinical advice for diagnosis and treatment of any pores and skin condition.

Eczema, also acknowledged as atopic dermatitis, is a chronic pores and skin situation characterised with the aid of dry, itchy, and infected skin. It frequently develops in early childhood but can manifest at any age. The genuine cause is complicated and no longer thoroughly understood however entails a combination of genetic and environmental factors. Flare-ups can be brought about by means of a range of irritants, allergens, stress, and pores and skin infections.

Here's a short information on managing eczema:

1. Moisturize Regularly: Apply fragrance-free moisturizers at once after bathing to lock moisture in the skin. Ointments and creams are extra positive than lotions.

2. Gentle Skin Care: Use slight soap-free cleansers, avoid hot water when bathing or washing, and gently pat the skin dry.

3. Identify Triggers: Common triggers

encompass tough fabrics, detergents, smoke, perfumes, modifications in temperature, sweat, and stress. Identifying and fending off non-public triggers is crucial.

4. Avoid Scratching: Keep nails quick and think about wearing gloves at night. Scratching can worsen the pores and skin condition and lead to infections.

5. Medications: Topical corticosteroids can minimize inflammation at some stage in flare-ups. Other choices consist of calcineurin inhibitors, PDE4 inhibitors, or biologic drugs for extreme cases.

6. Wet Wraps: In acute phases, wet wraps with medicated lotions can be effective, as recommended with the aid of a healthcare provider.

7. Phototherapy: Exposure to UVA or UVB mild waves can be beneficial for some humans when preferred redress are not enough.

8. Diet: In some cases, positive ingredients may additionally trigger eczema. It's important to discover and keep away from these foods.

9. Stress Management: Since stress can motive flare-ups, strategies such as meditation, deep breathing exercises, or yoga may be helpful.

10. Regular Check-ups: Regular visits to a dermatologist can assist manipulate the circumstance effectively.

Remember, managing eczema is an ongoing process, and what works for one man or woman may also not work for another. It frequently requires a personalized method developed with a healthcare provider.

Courses Of Skin Rashes

Skin conditions can be influenced by a vast vary of factors, extensively classified into quite a few primary causes:

✓ Genetics: Certain skin conditions, like psoriasis and eczema, have a genetic predisposition and can run in families.

✓ Infections: Various organisms including bacteria (impetigo, cellulitis), viruses (warts, shingles), fungi (athlete's foot, ringworm), and parasites (scabies) can infect the skin.

✓ Allergens: Contact with allergens can spark conditions such as contact dermatitis and hives.

✓ Environmental Factors: Exposure to sun, wind, cold, and chemical compounds can purpose stipulations like sunburn, rosacea, or chemical burns.

✓ Immune System Dysfunction: Abnormal immune responses can lead to prerequisites like psoriasis or lupus pores and skin manifestations.

✓ Lifestyle Choices: Poor nutrition, lack of sleep, smoking, and excessive stress can have an effect on pores and skin health, leading to conditions like acne.

✓ Hormonal Changes: Fluctuations in hormones, as viewed in puberty, pregnancy, or menopause, can trigger prerequisites such as acne or melasma.

Creams and physique lotions are applied to the pores and skin to moisturize, protect, and sometimes deal with unique skin conditions. However, in some instances, they can make a contribution to skin conditions:

✓ Allergic Reactions: Some people may also be allergic to ingredients in these products, main to contact dermatitis, characterized by way of redness, itching, and rash.

✓ Clogged Pores: Heavy lotions can block pores, causing acne or exacerbating prerequisites like folliculitis where hair follicles turn out to be inflamed.

✓Irritation: Components like fragrances, dyes, or preservatives can irritate sensitive skin, inflicting redness, stinging, or itching.

✓Incorrect Use: Using a product no longer acceptable to your pores and skin type (e.g., using an oil-based cream on oily skin) can lead to problems like greasiness or acne.

It's key to pick out products suitable for your skin type and to behavior a patch test earlier than full utility to reduce the danger of destructive reactions. Skin stipulations might also end result from a single aspect or a mixture of them, and their motives can frequently be multifactorial.

How To Control Their Growth

To control the growth of skin conditions, which include a number of types of pores and skin growths and acne, there are countless techniques and remedies available:

Skin Growth Control:

• Moles: Generally innocent but can be eliminated for cosmetic motives or if they exhibit signs and symptoms of change.

• Lentigines (Sun Spots): Can be treated with bleaching creams containing retinoids or hydroquinone.

• Seborrheic Keratosis': Usually harmless however can be removed if they reason irritation.

• Skin Tags: Can be eliminated with the aid of a healthcare issuer if favored for beauty reasons.

• Sebaceous Hyperplasia: Removal for beauty purposes is an option.

Cherry Angioma: Typically benign and may additionally not require treatment until for aesthetic reasons.

Acne Control:

• Home Remedies: Tea tree oil, apple cider vinegar, inexperienced tea, aloe Vera, and honey-cinnamon masks can help reduce irritation and battle acne-causing bacteria.

Topical Treatments: Over-the-counter

merchandise with benzoyl peroxide, salicylic acid, or adapalene can be advantageous for moderate acne.

• Prescription Medications: Dermatologists may prescribe topical retinoids, antibiotics, or oral medicines like isotretinoin for severe acne.

• Lifestyle Changes: Good simple skin care practices, keeping off irritants, the usage of noncomedogenic products, defending pores and skin from the sun, and fending off friction on acne-prone areas can help control acne.

It's essential to seek advice from with a dermatologist to decide the most appropriate cure diagram primarily based on the unique skin circumstance and character needs.

Common reasons of skin growths encompass more than a few factors such as genetics, solar exposure, hormonal changes, and aging. Some common sorts of pores and skin growths and their motives are:

• Actinic Keratosis: Caused via chronic sun exposure, main to rough, scaling spots on the pores and skin that are often tender.

• Epidermoid Cyst: Commonly determined on the face, back, or legs, these cysts result from blocked hair follicles and can be surgically removed when inflamed.

• Lipoma: A benign fatty growth that can boost below the pores and skin and is more common in men and women with a family records of lipomas.

• Sebaceous Hyperplasia: Seen in sufferers with oily skin due to an extra of oil glands, often acting as round "doughnuts" with a central depression.

Seborrheic Keratosis: Inherited lesions that generally appear after the age of 30 and are greater common in middle-aged and older individuals.

• Wart: Caused by way of a papillomavirus infection, warts are benign growths that may additionally require redress like laser therapy or medicines to increase the immune system.

These skin growths can differ in appearance and characteristics, with some being harmless whilst others may require scientific interest or removal for beauty reasons. It's vital to consult a dermatologist for ideal diagnosis and cure primarily based on the specific kind of pores and skin growth.

Risk factors for growing skin growths include:

- Genetics: A family records of pores and skin cancer or moles increases the likelihood of growing skin growths.

- Fair skin: Individuals with truthful skin, light hair, and light eyes are greater prone to skin growths, as they have much less melanin to protect their skin from UV radiation.

- Sun exposure: Exposure to UV radiation from the sun or tanning beds is a sizable danger issue for pores and skin growths, along with skin cancer.

- Age: The risk of developing pores and skin growths increases with age, as skin becomes extra susceptible to damage from the environment and herbal aging processes.

- Immune system: People with weakened immune systems, such as those with

HIV/AIDS or those taking immunosuppressant drugs after an organ transplant, are at expanded chance for skin growths.

- Exposure to toxic substances: Exposure to supplies like arsenic can expand the chance of pores and skin growths, consisting of skin cancer.

- Personal history of skin cancer: Individuals who have had pores and skin most cancers earlier than are at a higher chance of developing additional pores and skin growths.

- Moles: Having many moles or unusual moles known as dysplastic nevi increases the danger of skin growths.

- Exposure to radiation: People who have acquired radiation therapy for pores and skin stipulations might also have an expanded risk of skin cancer, in particular basal telephone carcinoma.

- Living at high altitudes: Elevation will increase the intensity of UV radiation, which can make contributions to the improvement of skin growths.

It's fundamental to be aware of these danger factors and take gorgeous measures to shield your skin, such as the usage of sunscreen, sporting protective clothing, and warding off immoderate solar exposure. Regular pores and skin examinations and early detection can additionally help in managing and treating skin growths.

Why Always Pimple And Eczema On My Body

Pimples are a frequent skin condition that occurs when hair follicles underneath the pores and skin turn out to be clogged with excess sebum and useless pores and skin cells, leading to infection of the hair follicles. This blockage can result in a range of kinds of lesions, which includes blackheads, whiteheads, pimples, papules, pustules, nodules, cysts, and abscesses. Acne is the most frequent skin disease in the United States, affecting 80% of the population at some factor in life.

It's essential to differentiate between pimples and other skin prerequisites that may resemble pimples. Conditions like perioral dermatitis, hidradenitis supputative, folliculitis, rosacea, staph infections, and even pores and skin most cancers can current with signs and symptoms similar to pimples but require unique treatments. Proper prognosis with the aid of a dermatologist is indispensable to determine the suitable remedy for these conditions.

Understanding the reasons and types of pimples lesions is necessary for superb management. Factors like extra oil production, dead skin cellphone buildup, bacterial increase in pores, hormonal changes, genetics, medications, and environmental factors can make a contribution to the improvement of acne. Treatment choices for pimples vary from topical preparations and antibiotics for slight cases to distortion for extreme acne. While zits are a common manifestation of pimples triggered with the aid of clogged hair follicles, it is essential to think about different pores and skin stipulations that may additionally mimic pimples to make sure accurate prognosis and gorgeous treatment.

There are several types of pimples, each

with awesome characteristics and severity levels:

✓ Blackheads: Open come-dunes filled with extra oil and dead pores and skin cells that show up black on the floor of the skin.

✓ Whiteheads: Closed come-dunes the place oil and pores and skin cells block a hair follicle barring opening, resulting in a white bump.

✓ Papules: Inflamed come-dunes forming small crimson or red bumps on the skin, regularly touchy to touch.

✓ Pustules: Inflamed zits reminiscent of whiteheads with a pink ring round them, typically stuffed with white or yellow pus.

✓ Nodules: Large, firm, inflamed bumps deep inside the skin that are regularly painful and may require dermatological treatment.

✓ Cysts: Large, pus-filled lesions similar to boils that can be painful and lead to scarring if not handled promptly.

These different sorts of acne can range from mild (blackheads and whiteheads) to reasonable (papules and pustules) to extreme (nodules and cysts). Proper diagnosis through a dermatologist is quintessential for identifying the terrific cure based totally on the kind and severity of acne lesions.

Treatment and remedies for acne can

consist of each herbal home remedies and conventional treatments. Some popular home treatments include:

✓ Tea tree oil: Apply diluted tea tree oil at once to pimples to combat infection and acne-causing bacteria.

✓ Apple cider vinegar: Dilute apple cider vinegar and practice it to the skin to assist decrease infection and fight acne-causing bacteria.

✓ Green tea: Apply green tea extract or brewed inexperienced tea to the skin to help battle infection and limit sebum production.

✓ Aloe Vera: Apply aloe Vera gel to the pores and skin to soothe and moisturize the skin, supporting to decrease inflammation and irritation.

✓ Honey and cinnamon: Mix honey and cinnamon to create a masks and observe it to the skin to help fight inflammation and reduce acne.

Conventional treatments for pimples include:

Topical creams and gels: Over-the-counter products containing components like benzoyl peroxide, salicylic acid, or adapalene can assist minimize acne.

Prescription medications: Dermatologists may also prescribe topical retinoids, antibiotics, or different medications to treat acne.

Lifestyle changes: Avoiding touching pimples, deciding on the right cleanser, and the use of oil-free pores and skin care merchandise can assist reduce acne.

It's vital to notice that the effectiveness of these remedies may additionally differ from character to person, and it's constantly satisfactory to consult a dermatologist for personalized treatment recommendations.

How Some body Creams Courses Rashes

Creams and physique lotions are applied to the pores and skin to moisturize, protect, and sometimes deal with unique skin conditions. However, in some instances, they can make a contribution to skin conditions:

✓ Allergic Reactions: Some people may also be allergic to ingredients in these products, main to contact dermatitis, characterized by way of redness, itching, and rash.

✓ Clogged Pores: Heavy lotions can block pores, causing acne or exacerbating prerequisites like folliculitis where hair follicles turn out to be inflamed.

✓ Irritation: Components like fragrances, dyes, or preservatives can irritate sensitive skin, inflicting redness, stinging, or itching.

✓Incorrect Use: Using a product no longer acceptable to your pores and skin type (e.g., using an oil-based cream on oily skin) can lead to problems like greasiness or acne. It's key to pick out products suitable for your skin type and to behavior a patch test earlier than full utility to reduce the danger of destructive reactions.

Body lotions make a contribution to skin conditions with the aid of moisturizing the skin, enhancing hydration, and aiding the pores and skin micro-biome. These lotions incorporate emollients that soften the skin and assist keep its herbal pH balance, which is fundamental for a wholesome skin micro-biome. The lipid composition of the skin is superior by means of body lotions, main to upgrades in pores and skin health measures like dryness, hydration, and skin cohesively. Additionally, certain micro organism found in the skin, like Staphylococcus epidermis, can be extended by body lotions, promotion really helpful effects on the skin. Emollients in physique lotions are particularly advisable for stipulations like eczema and psoriasis, offering alleviation from dryness, cracking, and scaling. They shape a shielding barrier on the skin's surface, preventing moisture loss and enhancing comfort for persons with touchy or dry skin. However, it is fundamental to select merchandise cautiously to avoid viable irritants and allergens that should irritate pores and skin conditions. In essence, physique lotions play a good sized function in keeping pores and skin fitness through improving hydration, helping the pores and skin micro-biome, and bettering the standard condition of the skin.

Common Food That Courses Skin Rashes

Some frequent foods that can result in pores and skin condition problems include:

° High Glycemic Index (GI) Foods: Foods like white bread, white pasta, potatoes, and sugary baked items with a high GI can increase the chances of creating pimples and trigger premature tissue growing older thru a technique called glaciation.

° Processed Meats: Processed meats such

as bacon or hotdogs contain high ranges of nitrates and sodium, which can lead to inflammation, wrinkles, untimely aging, dryness, and collagen harm in the skin.

° Dairy Products: Cow's milk and dairy merchandise made from cow's milk have been linked to pores and skin stipulations like acne and psoriasis due to their potential to bring up insulin tiers and make bigger sebum production, contributing to pimples development.

° Alcohol: Alcohol is a diuretic that can dehydrate the skin, main to dryness and accelerating the skin's ageing process, resulting in premature fine strains and wrinkles.

° Tomatoes, Citrus Fruits, Foods Containing Nickel, and Spices: These meals can motive skin irritations in people sensitive to materials like Balsam of Peru, citrus peel, nickel, or certain spices like cinnamon and cloves. Allergic reactions to these foods can manifest as redness, swelling, rashes, or itchiness on the skin.

It's essential to be conscious of these meals if you have touchy pores and skin or are prone to skin conditions. Consulting with a healthcare expert or dermatologist can help pick out particular dietary triggers for your skin troubles and guide you on making appropriate dietary adjustments.

CHAPTER 3

Preventing Skin Rashes

Prevention for pores and skin prerequisites can vary depending on the unique condition. Here are some typical tips to forestall a range of pores and skin conditions:

Wash your face daily: Use a gentle cleanser and water to remove dirt, oil, and impurities.

> Moisturize: Apply a moisturizer to preserve your pores and skin hydrated and protect it from environmental factors.

> Avoid allergens: Stay away from foods,

cosmetics, or different products that purpose allergic reactions on your skin.

> Avoid harsh chemicals: Steer clear of harsh chemical compounds or other irritants that can injury your skin.

> Sleep well: Ensure you get at least 7 hours of sleep each night to guide pores and skin health.

> Stay hydrated: Drink masses of water to keep your skin hydrated and hold its overall health.

> Eat a balanced diet: Consume a weight loss program wealthy in fruits, vegetables, complete grains, and lean proteins to support skin health.

> Protect your skin: Shield your skin from

immoderate cold, heat, and wind to forestall damage.

> Sun protection: Use sunscreen, hats, and shielding clothing to guard your pores and skin from the sun's dangerous UV rays.

> Maintain correct hygiene: Wash your hands regularly and keep away from sharing non-public objects to forestall the spread of infectious skin conditions.

For unique skin conditions, additional prevention techniques may also be necessary. For example, for acne prevention, keep away from excessive glycemic index foods and restriction dairy products. For eczema, keep away from viable triggers like nickel, positive spices, and meals additives. Consult a healthcare professional or dermatologist for customized prevention techniques based on your unique skin condition.

Some frequent skin stipulations that can be avoided include:

> Acne: Prevent acne with the aid of washing your face each day with a mild cleanser, the usage of moisturizer, heading off high-glycemic foods, and preserving right hygiene practices.

> Eczema: Reduce eczema flare-ups by means of warding off triggers like positive foods, using moisturizers, and incorporating omega-3 fats, zinc, and

nutrition E in your diet.

> Psoriasis: Prevent psoriasis flare-ups by maintaining a healthful weight loss program rich in entire grains and low in unhealthy fat and sugars, defending your pores and skin from environmental factors, and managing stress levels.

> Skin Aging: Protect your pores and skin from excessive solar exposure, keep away from excessive glycemic index foods, restriction alcohol consumption, and preserve proper hydration to forestall untimely growing older of the skin.

> Sunburn: Prevent sunburn by using the use of sunscreen, sporting protective clothing, and limiting solar exposure for

the duration of height hours.

> Lice: Avoid sharing non-public objects like hairbrushes or hats to prevent the unfold of lice.

> Pemphigus and Pemphigoid: These autoimmune skin prerequisites may also not be preventable but can be managed with medical treatment.

> Lichen Planus: While the purpose is no longer fully understood, averting potential triggers like positive medicinal drugs or infections may also assist forestall flare-ups.

> Erythema Multi-forme: This circumstance can be caused via infections or medications; stopping these triggers can

help reduce the danger of creating erythema multi-forme.

By following acceptable skincare routines, maintaining a wholesome diet, protecting your skin from environmental factors, and managing stress levels, you can substantially limit the threat of developing a number skin conditions.

Therapy For Managing Skin Conditions

Therapies for various skin conditions can include a range of treatments depending on the specific condition. Here are some frequent cures for skin conditions:

> Antihistamines: Used to treat allergic reactions and itching associated with skin conditions.

> Medicated Creams and Ointments: Topical treatments that can assist control a range of skin problems like eczema, psoriasis, and acne.

> Biologics: Used for treating extreme pores and skin conditions like psoriasis, biologics work via focused on unique components of the immune machine involved in the ailment process.

> Phototherapy (Light Therapy): Utilizes

ultraviolet light to efficaciously treat pores and skin ailments such as psoriasis, vitiligo, eczema, actinic keratosis, acne, scleroderma, and exclusive sorts of pores and skin cancers. It consists of techniques like phototherapy, photodynamic therapy, and photochemotherapy.

> Probiotics: Adjunct therapy with probiotics (oral or topical) has been discovered positive in managing pimples by directly impacting the skin's microbiome.

> Herbal Medicine: Some natural marketers like tea tree oil and barberry extract have proven beneficial results in managing skin prerequisites like acne.

> Zinc Supplementation: Oral zinc supplementation has been studied for its efficacy in treating acne, with some studies displaying nice consequences over placebo.

> Gugulipid: An extract of gum guggul that has been compared to oral tetracycline for treating nodulocystic acne, displaying improvement in pimples lesions.

These healing procedures can be nice in managing a range of pores and skin conditions, but it's critical to seek advice from with a healthcare provider or dermatologist to determine the most suitable cure diagram based on the particular condition and character needs.

Some choice remedies for skin conditions include:

Herbal Medicine: Herbal redress like tea tree oil, barberry extract, and gugulipid have shown really helpful results in managing pores and skin stipulations like acne.

Probiotics: Probiotics, whether or not taken orally or applied topically, can play a position in managing pimples via at once impacting the skin's microbiome.

Traditional Chinese Medicine (TCM): TCM remedies are sought by way of sufferers for a number of skin prerequisites and can encompass herbal

treatments and dietary modifications.

Mind/Body Interventions: Practices like meditation, yoga, and stress administration methods can assist enhance ordinary pores and skin fitness by means of reducing stress stages that may exacerbate positive skin conditions.

Dietary Modifications: Adjusting one's food plan to encompass or knock out specific foods recognised to set off or irritate pores and skin prerequisites can be an fine alternative therapy.

Home UV Phototherapy Systems: These structures may also enhance treatment adherence for positive pores and skin stipulations like psoriasis but ought to be

used below medical supervision.

Vascular Lasers and Intense Pulse Lights: While now not currently advocated for inflammatory skin diseases, these remedies may have workable advantages for sure pores and skin conditions when used appropriately.

Low-Level Light Treatment: Another structure of phototherapy that might also have functions in treating a number of skin disorders.

Alternative healing procedures can provide extra selections for managing skin conditions, but it's quintessential to consult with a healthcare provider or dermatologist before starting any alternative treatment to make certain protection and effectiveness, specifically when combining them with traditional scientific treatments.

Recommendations

The suggestions for skin stipulations include a number preventive measures and treatment options to keep pores and skin health. Here is a precis primarily based on the provided search results:

* Prevention Techniques: Preventing skin stipulations includes practices like

washing your face every day with a mild cleanser, using moisturizer, heading off allergens, harsh chemicals, and irritants, getting adequate sleep, staying hydrated, ingesting a balanced diet, and defending your pores and skin from environmental factors like excessive temperatures.

* Treatment Options: Treatment for skin prerequisites can encompass antihistamines, medicated creams and ointments, biologics, phototherapy, probiotics, natural medicine, zinc supplementation, and gugulipid. These treatments can assist control a number skin problems like acne, eczema, psoriasis, and more.

* Alternative Therapies: Alternative healing procedures for skin conditions may additionally involve natural medicine, probiotics, usual Chinese remedy (TCM), mind/body interventions like meditation and yoga, dietary modifications, domestic UV phototherapy systems, vascular lasers, and low-level mild treatment.

* Dietary Interventions: Diet plays a function in dermatology; dietary modifications can impact the route of pores and skin illnesses like zits and serve as a preventive measure for stipulations such as pores and skin most cancers and ageing of the skin. Dermatologists may also propose dietary changes to enhance

skin fitness and control positive conditions.

* Skin Health Practices: To preserve healthful skin, it's vital to wear protective gear when needed, smooth cuts or scrapes right now with soap and water, defend against sunburn with excellent clothing and sunscreen, exercise properly hygiene by washing fingers frequently, and use slight cleansers when bathing.

By following these recommendations on prevention techniques, therapy options, alternative therapies, dietar interventions, and standard pores and skin health practices, humans can efficiently manage more than a few skin conditions and promote normal skin health.

CAUSES OF TEXTURED SKIN

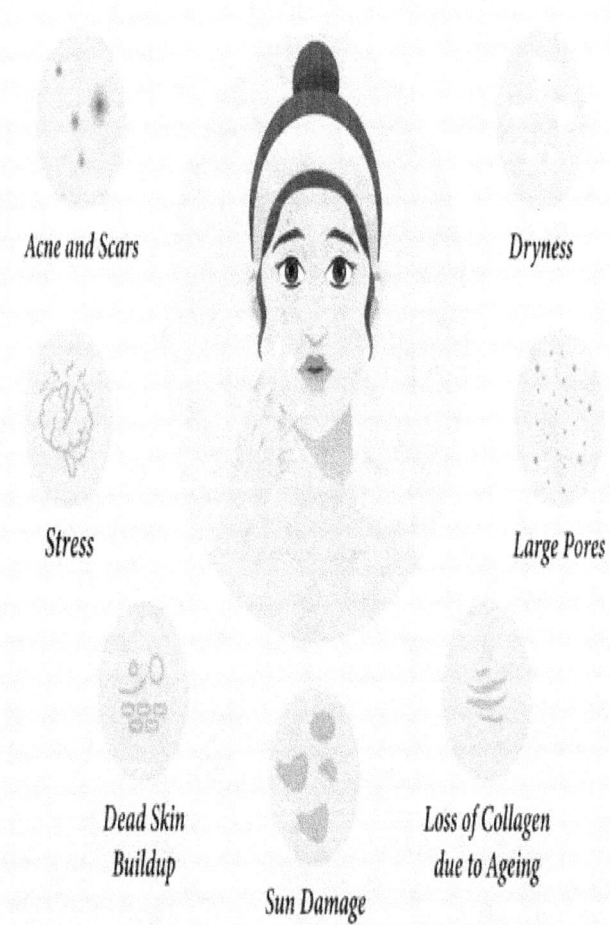